Even

You

Can Be

Healthy!

3-Step Guide for Busy People
Plus Easy Recipes

Ann Prospero

First Printing, 2013
ISBN 978-0-615-66643-3
Library of Congress Registration Number Txu 1-830-866

*To George W. Newton, who realized
how much we all need this book today*

"Keep your thoughts positive because your thoughts become your words. Keep your words positive because your words become your behavior. Keep your behavior positive because your behavior becomes your habits. Keep your habits positive because your habits become your values. Keep your values positive because your values become your destiny."

Mahatma Gandhi

Acknowledgements

A number of talented individuals have contributed freely to this book, making it highly useful and dependable. The goal of this book is to keep it simple so that anyone can have a healthy life.

All of the contributors have helped make this book, *Even You Can Be Healthy!*, simple-to-use, and it will show you how to bring sane eating, exercise, and stress relief into your lives in today's extraordinarily busy world. The recipes alone contribute to a fit body that maintains a healthy weight. You'll see it all inside!

Contributors

Nutritionist
Kara Mitchell, MS, RD/LD, ACSM-RCEP, is currently a Dietitian, Exercise Physiologist and Wellness Manager at the Duke Health & Fitness Center, Durham, NC. She gladly reviewed the sections on nutrition as well as the sections of recipes. Her suggestions have been implemented in this book and her judgments have helped make this book trustworthy.

Copyeditors
Elaine Bauman, Marcia L. Tuttle, and **Carol Wills,** each is extremely qualified and experienced. They have helped make this book consistent and reliable.

Recipe Testers
The Recipe Testers came from as far away as Australia and the United Kingdom. Most were from the United States: North Carolina, including Durham and Chapel Hill, and New Jersey. Some of the best contributions came from those recipe testers who don't usually cook their own meals. They saw that many of these recipes needed changing or deleting altogether, making them better for you.

Emma Allan, United Kingdom, lived as a child in Australia, Asia, and Europe. Later she gave up her corporate career in marketing and was surprised to discover that food was her true passion. She loves nothing more than trying out new recipes.

Carol Cantrell, a North Carolina teacher and experienced cook, grew up in Stephens, Arkansas, the younger daughter of two fine cooks. She has enjoyed the "best" restaurants and food all over the world, including in five cities in China.

Meredith Downing, Durham, NC, is a recent graduate of Louisiana State University with a Bachelor of Science in Kinesiology, and a concentration in Fitness Studies. Meredith loves all types of food, especially spicy foods and seafood.

Angela Eberts, Chapel Hill, NC. Her cooking is usually most appreciated by her husband and two children. She works at Duke University's Fuqua School of Business as an Associate Program Director for the Master of Management Studies program. She catered in Chicago and demonstrated recipes and products at A Southern Season in Chapel Hill, NC.

Ann Hall, United Kingdom, has a food blog, Scrummy Suppers & Quirky Cakes, where she has uploaded the two recipes she tested from *Even You Can Be Healthy!* She is an Irish-born "mum" of two and loves to cook. Currently a research scientist for malaria, she is working towards becoming involved in food publishing and recipe testing as a new career.

Nicole Hayward, Melbourne, Australia, is self employed and works from home, where she has found a new passion—to be a wonderful cook. She loves trying new recipes and being creative with them.

Matt Lardie, Durham, NC. He works as a cheese maker and freelance food writer. He is involved in the local sustainable agriculture community and is a strong proponent of healthy home cooking (see Green Eats Blog).

Kathryn Cain Parkins, Durham, NC, is a very accomplished organist and church musician who comes from a long line of people who don't cook. She says, "Instead of leaning about practical things like cooking, I spent all of my time practicing." She was raised on the freshest TV dinners that the 1950s produced. She was eager to try the recipes for this book as they were easy to follow and produced results that made her realize the truth that, "Anyone that can read can cook."

Linda Prospero, Princeton, NJ, spent her career as a journalist for newspapers and international wire services and her work has appeared in publications ranging from *The New York Times* and *Los Angeles Times* to the *Times of India*. Her real passion however is Italy—its landscape, art, music, culture, and especially its food. She enjoys sharing that love with friends and family and is the author of the popular blog, *Ciao Chow Linda, ciaochowlinda.blogspot.com/*

Ruth Porter, Durham, NC, is an artisan baker and student of cooking at "Chef's Choice" classes at Johnson & Wales, Charlotte, NC. "I learned to cook from the early Julia Child shows. My grandmother taught me to bake bread while I was a teenager. Today, all of the bread we eat is home-made."

Steven Risi, Durham, NC, has a BS in Health Fitness, is a Certified Trainer with the American College of Sports Medicine, and is an Exercise Specialist at the Duke Diet and Fitness Center and Duke Health and Fitness Center at the Center for Living. Steven's food interests include custom seasoning, vegetable pita pizzas, spicy recipes (chicken), and Mexican dinners.

Carol Wills, Durham, NC, served as a copy editor of *Even You Can Be Healthy!* and was with the Durham based *Independent Weekly* and Duke University. She also served as a Recipe Tester. Born in Tennessee, Carol grew up on a typical Appalachian-style diet of beans and cornbread seasoned with bacon grease and sugary fruit pies with crusts made from Crisco. She has became aware that a plant-based diet, free from animal fats and excessive sweetening, was going to make the difference for her between a reasonably healthy old age and chronic illness.

Jean Wilson, Durham, NC, born in Mississippi, grew up as an army brat and studied French at the University of North Carolina at Chapel Hill. Jean's culinary experiences range from enjoying Southern cooking from the bounty of her grandparents' farm, as well as Japanese and French cuisine, when her father was stationed in Kokura, Japan, and Poitiers, France.

Contents

Healthy Eating Contents
Spring and Summer

Fall and Winter

Celebrations!

More Healthy, Easy Recipes

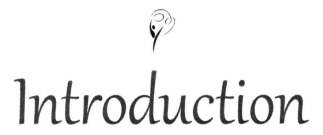

Introduction

Even **You** Can Be Healthy!

Beginners Guide to Great Health

This book is for all of you who want to be healthier and to have a better quality of life but don't really know where to begin. And this book is for those of you who don't have the time or energy or money or ability to make the move to what you imagine is a more demanding way of living and eating.

Actually you'll see that living a healthy life will release all the stored up energy and vitality you have hidden in you. You'll begin to do the things you want to do—gardening, wood working, hiking in the woods, cooking, playing sports, feeling good about yourself. You'll be able to attend the worship services of your choice, work regularly at your job, volunteer, and go out with friends. And you save money when your evermore frequent visits to doctors' offices become unnecessary.

Your first and most important step to leading a healthy lifestyle is to make the decision to do just that.

My goal is to help you make living a healthier lifestyle easy and achievable. We're going to live a long and good life in as easy a way as possible. We'll end up as stronger people than we ever thought possible. Here comes your part: Your first and most important step to leading a healthy lifestyle is to make the decision to do just that. When you do, this book will make whatever changes are necessary to become healthy easier to do than you thought.

There are shortcuts here that you may not have known about. I'll give you a basic rundown on exercise and how you can bring it easily into your everyday life, on stress relief and how to find it a few moments at a time, and on healthy eating with simple-to-make recipes along with a quick course on nutrition.

This book sets you up to lead a healthy lifestyle in ways that even you can do. So let's begin this journey to health together. Let's leave behind those diseases that lurk underneath a lifestyle with no exercise, without relief of your stress, with the kinds of foods that clog your arteries and lead to obesity.

When you become healthy, you'll be almost free from obesity, diabetes, high blood pressure, heart disease, cancer, depression, and many other diseases linked to unhealthy lifestyles. For example, a National Institutes of Health/AARP study has shown that leading a healthy lifestyle may reduce the risk factors of Type 2 diabetes by about 80 percent among men and women aged 50 to 71. (Think of the medical bills!) You can do it—simply and easily. This book shows you how.

Here you'll find simple techniques to bring into your everyday life the three basic steps toward great health—exercise, stress relief, and healthy eating. They will become a natural part of your life because you'll feel so much better, mentally and physically. And you deserve it.

Chapter 1

Why Bother?

A Healthy Lifestyle

for Increased Energy and Stamina, Clearer Mind, and Better Quality of Life

Our lives these days are filled with activities, responsibilities, and things that must be done—now! We don't exercise. We probably don't get enough sleep. And we don't eat right because we don't have the time to cook and because we think it's easier to go out to eat or to pick up a packaged meal. We combine eating with meetings and work in our attempts to save time and energy.

Yet paying attention to a healthy lifestyle pays dividends far beyond the time and effort expended. The cornerstones of a healthy lifestyle are:

- exercise,

- rest and stress relief, and, above all,

- healthy eating.

Results are almost immediate. When we engage in even a minimally healthy lifestyle, right away we gain more energy, feel good about our lifestyle and ourselves, have longer life spans, and are free from diseases associated with unhealthy living. And, best of all, we are more in control of our lives.

When we're young, by following a healthy lifestyle, we can help prevent having a lifetime full of disease and disability. We may think those diseases are just an inconvenience, but they are truly dreadful—loss of limbs, blindness, loss of the use of our minds, even early loss of life. As we age, this is especially true.

It's our decision to become healthy. By following the simple steps described in this book, you'll soon see that, yes, you can do it.

Make the Decision

Developing a healthy lifestyle requires change. It requires breaking harmful old habits. It requires making decisions instead of automatically moving the way we've always moved, relieving stress the way we've always relieved stress, and eating the way we've always eaten.

No longer will we stop by the bakery or coffee shop to buy cupcakes. Nor will we pick up a quick meal bought at a fast food restaurant because we think it's easier and saves time. Nor will we eat all the goodies brought to us as gifts. No longer will we succumb to the many unhealthy lures and temptations out there.

Developing a healthy lifestyle requires change.
It requires breaking harmful old habits.

We'll discover that just sitting behind a computer screen can be harmful, though getting up several times a day and moving around will help you to discover health. We'll turn off the television and put down late-night work because we know we'll be refreshed, alert, and more productive the next day when we get a good night's sleep.

Soon the old way of living will feel wrong and the new way will be so rewarding that it seems natural, easy, and good. Because we'll feel much better, we're no longer tempted by harmful, old habits. We'll develop healthy, new habits.

Every Day

Our new, strong, vibrant life begins when we decide to be good to our bodies. First, we'll stock our kitchens with healthy food so that all our snacks are healthy. We won't be tempted to eat chips just because they're handy. And we'll begin to ask ourselves, "Am I truly hungry?" Every day.

We'll decide to order healthy food at a restaurant or fast food outlet instead of the all-too-tempting fried foods and beckoning desserts. Every day.

We'll decide to exercise by getting outside for a walk, going to the gym, or exercising at home. Regular exercise as well as healthy eating will become a vital part of our lives. Every day.

Worth the Effort

Trust me. You can teach yourself to do these things. This is not a quick weight-loss diet or fast lifestyle change. Positive results will be gradual. As our lifestyle improves, so will our mental health, physical health, and ability to think clearly. Weight loss and a healthier body and mind will follow. And gradually, it all will become easy.

Chapter 2

Move!

Exercise in Your Everyday Life

Along, vital life. Good health. Weight loss. Mood enhancement. Firm bodies. These benefits don't come just from eating and drinking right. In fact, you won't get these benefits unless you move your body *and* practice healthy eating.

Moving, or exercise, directs the calories and nutrients you get from all the good food you eat and the liquid you drink to the benefit of your changing body. Exercise helps you lose weight. It gradually firms the body that you thought was going to flab. It fights depression.

Exercise along with healthy eating and drinking will benefit both your body *and* your mind. Your outlook on life improves when you exercise, and your body improves as well.

> *"The number of Americans who are overweight or obese is 66.5 percent .... That's astonishing," says Lewis Bowling.*

It's a circle—when your body improves, so does your attitude. Your exercising body affects your emotions, and your improving emotions affect your physical being, and both your emotions and your improving body inspire you to eat healthily and not to binge on high-sugar, high-fat, or high-salt foods. That alone is an excellent reason to bring regular exercise into your life.

Without exercise, those calories you ingest, no matter what they are and where they come from, will turn to fat. With exercise, your calories will turn to muscle. Think about it:

"The number of Americans who are overweight or obese is 66.5 percent, according to the Statistical Abstract of the United States. That's astonishing," says fitness columnist Lewis Bowling in the *Durham Herald Sun* and instructor at Duke University and North Carolina Central University. "That statistic is primarily due to lack of exercise," continues Bowling.

The consequences of being overweight include diabetes, heart disease, sleep disorders, and low energy levels among many other disorders, including depression. Yet by exercising even the minimum amount, you increase your stamina, endurance, energy levels, and emotional well being. Just by moving, you improve your overall health.

Bringing Exercise into Your Day-to-Day Life

You can begin by taking just 2000 steps, such as walking for 20 minutes or around one or two blocks near your house, every day. Or by using an exercise machine such as Nu-Step where you sit and move your legs and arms. Or do some wall push ups by standing or sitting in front of a wall, reaching your straight arms to touch the wall, and pushing back and forth.

Whatever you choose, begin gradually. You'll be surprised at how fast you improve. When you move more briskly, you'll also curb your appetite and cravings.

More importantly, you'll discover that if you can get outside or begin to move your body, you'll change the narrow, inward focus of your life. You'll lighten up, you'll be more positive, and you'll feel confident that you can do it all.

It's as if the world has opened and you've begun to participate. As you begin to take control of your life by exercising and making other healthful changes, your attitude toward your life will change and become more positive. And you'll begin to embrace life rather than dread the way you look and feel.

If You Are New to Exercise

If you currently have a sedentary lifestyle or you've avoided exercise because you don't like it or you think it's too much trouble, commit yourself anyway to some kind of exercise every day.

It's important, though, to find what works for you. If you don't like an exercise routine, you won't do it.

- There are many kinds of exercise to choose from—walking, climbing stairs instead of taking the elevator, cleaning the house by sweeping or vacuuming, yard work like raking or stooping to plant vegetables or flowers, attending a gym on a regular basis, hiking in the woods or around the mall. Exercise includes whatever you do to move your body, even if you can't stand up. (If you're starting a brand new exercise program, make sure your doctor approves what you've chosen as your exercise.)

- At first exercise two or three times a week. Start out with ten minutes of movement such as walking or even cleaning the house or raking the yard or doing wall pushups. If you're aiming for thirty minutes of exercise a day, and that's a good start, you can do it in ten-minute blocks, three times a day. Just get moving!

- When you start, you probably won't have much stamina. That will come to you a little at a time as you exercise. Build up your stamina bit by bit, exercising every day. Then exercise a little bit more. You'll be amazed at how quickly stamina sneaks up on you.

- Every day add a few more minutes of exercise until you are moving thirty minutes and then eventually an hour a day. Break your exercise sessions into small blocks of time.

- You can easily achieve your exercise goal by parking at the end of the parking lot and walking to the front door, by taking breaks frequently from your desk at the office and walking around for a few minutes, or by holding a hand weight and do-ing a few curls as you read your email or are sitting in a chair.

- Don't become sedentary by sitting at the computer or in front of the TV for hours on end. Even if you've exercised in the morning or plan on exercising in the early evening, it's impor-tant that you make an effort to get up from your desk and do something—walk to the water cooler, do some deep knee bends at your desk. Be sure that you move your body as often as every hour. Try setting a timer, either on your computer or smart phone to remind you to get up and move on a regular basis.

- Make stretching a part of your exercise regimen. You can stretch your legs and arms after you warm up by walking or moving for a while. Some people stretch after their aerobic or strengthening exercise session. You'll feel your muscles stretch, and each time you do it, they'll stretch a little further.

- Exercising in one burst of 30 to 60 minutes isn't enough. Frank-ly, you should accumulate activity throughout the day. Even if you've worked out that morning or the evening before, sitting all day is a form of sedentary lifestyle, leading to larger waists, higher blood pressure, higher levels of triglycerides, increased body inflammation, and lower levels of the good cholesterol. Take breaks to move and stretch to avoid all the problems of a sedentary lifestyle.

How It's Done by Real People

When I work at my computer, I set a timer for one hour. When it rings, I get up and walk around or do a set of exercises for a few minutes. That way I avoid getting stiff and sore, and I'm exercising throughout the day, feeling much more alert and able to continue my work.

Don't get discouraged. If you slack off or miss some of your planned workouts, simply begin again where you left off. Exercise is truly an important part of your healthy lifestyle. Because, when you exercise, you'll relieve any simmering depression, add joy to your life, make your brain sharper and work better, lower your blood pressure, and add to your better functioning overall.

Cost and Availability

If you can afford it, join a gym and commit to going several times a week. But that's not necessary. There are aerobics classes, often held for free or for very little money. Check the listings on the computer or watch the papers for times and places. Brisk walking and running in your neighborhood, in the mall, or on a jogging path will achieve the same results as a structured aerobics class—and it's free. And you can exercise freely at home. All you have to do it set a *regular* time to do it.

The equipment you need for an exercise program costs very little. Buy a set of light hand weights, if you wish, or use the weights that are actually free: canned goods or five-pound packages of sugar or flour in plastic shopping bags that you can lift by holding the handles.

The resistance bands and Thera-bands are cheap and available at sporting goods stores, big box stores, or online. Alternatively, you can use a thin towel or old stocking to perform the same routines by holding one end of the towel or stocking in one hand, anchor it with your feet or on a doorknob, and pull in the direction you are working on. You will be able to feel the muscles tightening.

Stretching is always free. After your workout, stretch those muscles you've been working by bending, raising up, pushing on muscles you've used.

Many books, commercial videos, or YouTube videos have demonstrations and instructions for exercising. In the library, you'll find numerous books and pamphlets on exercise. The government publications office has several booklets on exercise for free or a nominal fee.

Go to http://catalog.gpo.gov and type in Exercise and Physical Activity in the search space. Another good site is http://www.weboflife.nasa.gov/exerciseandaging/toc.html. These are excellent booklets to have on hand for reference.

Your Life

As you can see, there's no excuse for not exercising. For me personally, I find that if I get up early and go straight to my exercising routine without thinking and before I can make excuses for not exercising, I can do it easily and thoughtfully. It readies me for the day. For others, exercising when they get home from work or school is a good way to unwind. Whenever you choose to do it, exercise can make a huge difference in your life.

Find the best way and time for you to exercise. It's essential to your health that you commit to exercising, to calming yourself, and most importantly to healthy eating.

The reward is a far better lifestyle. You can do it!

Chapter 3

Calm and Peace

Moments at a Time

Reduce Stress

This step—finding calm in a crazy world—leads toward a healthy, long, vibrant life and is far more important than you may realize. You've committed to exercising and have seen that exercising can be a simple addition to your daily life. Soon you'll begin a eating a healthy diet as shown in Chapter 13, "Menus! Recipes!," pages 74-184, and in Chapter 8, "Healthy Eating Nutrition: Briefly," pages 45-55.

Here you'll learn how to find those precious moments of calm and peace in your hectic day. You may only find those moments for a few minutes, or even seconds, at a time. Even that tiny bit of time is a start. You'll discover during those short times that the calm and peace you have found will be with you to tap into the rest of the day or even when lying in bed at night.

How to Find Calm and Peace

If you're like most of us, your life is hectic. There are deadlines, people asking you to do things, and nothing going as planned. Maybe you don't feel well. Maybe you're making mistakes because you're overwhelmed. Maybe you're cranky and don't know why. What do you do about it?

Know that you deserve to quiet down and to find the calm and peace that's there inside you. Then do it.

There are several ways to become quiet:

- By sitting quietly by yourself even in a crowded space;

- By focusing just on sounds or colors or your breaths with no judgment;

- By paying attention only to what you are doing in the moment such as chewing your food, brushing your teeth, washing the dishes, riding in the car, or on any activity that you participate in during your day;

- And by learning the art of meditating.

When, for example, busy people feel stressed, they can concentrate on the sound of their steps every time they walk to and from their desks. Every time. That's just a few seconds at a time, but by doing these simple mindful tasks, they have calmed themselves and removed themselves from the bustle all around them.

Remember that the fact that you are alive is a gift. Enjoy it.

Finding your quiet space impacts your body and emotions. When you do find that quiet space, you're counteracting all the negative impacts of stress such as high blood pressure, impulsive eating, and the tendency to put off what is good for you.

Remember that the fact that you are alive is a gift. Enjoy it. Seek the beauty and laughter and joy that are part of life. It's out there somewhere. Look for it.

Methods of Calming Yourself

- **Allowing your mind to wander.** Sit or lie down in a quiet place for a few moments wherever you are. Do not think of all you have to do. Instead, imagine a scene or an event that you would love to be in. Think of the ocean, the forest, a ball game, or a garden, whatever makes you feel good. Do it for a few seconds or few minutes at a time. Your mind will wander. That's okay. Minds do that. Keep coming back gently to the pictures of what you love.

- **Deep breathing**. Something as simple as breathing can calm us and bring us peace. Noticing your breaths as they go in and out is a meditation technique; but here you are only going to breathe to soothe yourself in the midst of your busy, frantic life.

  - When you are anxious or worried, you probably begin to breathe shallowly. Counteract your body's impulse to tighten up by breathing deeply. The form of this practice is: breathe in through your nose, hold your breath, and breathe out through your nose or mouth.

  - Begin slowly with fewer than 10 breaths and repeat, working up to 10 breaths at a time. Then add up to 2 or 3 sets of 10 breaths each. Stop when or if you feel dizzy or faint. Your body will adjust to deep breathing in a few days.

  - The following is a deep breathing method that may calm you:

    - Either sit straight up or lie flat on your back.

    - Place your crossed hands loosely on your abdomen.

    - Inhale slowly and deeply through your nose for a count of at least 4. Your hands over your abdomen will rise as you breathe in and expand your lungs with air.

    - Hold your inhaled breath for a count of 4 or more.

    - Exhale the air very slowly through your nose, or mouth if necessary, for a count of 4 or more.

- **Music and relaxation tapes.** If you're too tired to concentrate, listening to calming music made especially for relaxing or popping in a relaxation CD is a passive way to relax. You can find these CDs on the Internet.

- **Yoga.** This is a mind-body exercise practice that combines deep breathing with stretching and a focus on postures. Yoga helps connect the body with the mind and is a meditation technique in itself. There are yoga DVDs that can be shown on a television set or computer screen, and classes are often available. If you choose to practice yoga, commit to it at least once a week.

Meditation Techniques

Research has shown that meditation truly manages stress and reduces pain. The idea behind meditation is to calm your body by focusing your mind for certain periods of time on something outside yourself.

Basically, the goal of meditation is to clear your mind of all the clutter that distracts us and all the worry that swirls around in our head. When you do that, you'll find calm and peace that lasts, and you'll find it overlaps with many areas of your life.

There are so many techniques for meditation available that you may be confused about which one to use. Your goal in meditation is to clear your mind of the turmoil and hubbub that crowd out all clear thinking. Keeping in mind that the goal is to clear your mind, you will discover eventually what works best for you.

Sample the following descriptions of meditation techniques, neither of which is at all difficult. Try these techniques for 10 to 20 minutes a day at a time that you've set aside for meditation. This is not a complete list, but it will get you started:

- **Mindfulness:** A popular technique.

  - One method of mindfulness meditation is to concentrate on your breaths as you breathe in and out. Feel the breath coming into your body. Hear the sounds of your breaths. As much as possible, be in the moment so that you notice only your breaths. Your mind will wander. Let it. When you can, turn your thoughts back to concentrating on your breathing.

- You can practice mindfulness throughout the day by focusing only on what you are doing at that moment, such as when you are brushing your teeth. Feel the pressure of the brush against your teeth and gums. What you are feeling means that you are alive.

- You can practice mindfulness when you are sitting quietly for a few minutes by listening to the sounds around you. Have no feelings about those sounds. Separate the sounds into different sounds. Maybe there's a clock ticking, the air conditioner blowing, a car traveling by on the street, birds singing outside the window. Just hear them. There should be no judgment about them. They are only sounds.

Usually mindfulness lasts only seconds before your mind begins to wander to the day's tasks. That's okay. Keep practicing. You'll get better at it.

- **Focus.** This practice is related to mindfulness.

  - Sit or lie down comfortably. Focus, either on a part of your body; on a flame; on an image; or on things such as sounds, waves, clouds, or nature.

  - You might repeat a sentence, a quote, or prayer that is meaningful to you. This repeated word, phrase, or sound is known as a mantra and is an aid to focusing your concentration away from distractions. You can repeat a mantra that can be as simple as the sound "Om," or another senseless word; or a deeply felt word or phrase related to spirituality.

Why Find Calm and Peace

Calming your mind and finding peace, whatever method you use, teaches the mind to stick to one object, action, or thought. Because the mind is usually restless, you're helping it become quiet, and when the mind is quiet, the body is quiet, too, working at its optimal levels.

To succeed in this truly necessary part of a healthy lifestyle, you need patience, some perseverance, and a belief that it will eventually work. You will succeed, progressing in small increments, just as you are doing with exercise and healthy eating.

The results of finding the calm and peace that are already inside you can lead to physical and mental health, along with enhanced powers of concentration, memory, intuition, and inner strength.

Chapter 4

Toward Health

Ways to Become Healthy through Good Diets

Healthy Eating—The Plan

Healthy eating, a significant part of your new healthy lifestyle, is really very simple. Follow these basic guidelines:

- Use lots of colorful vegetables and fruit, whether fresh, canned, or frozen.

- Use mostly "good" fats such as olive oil and other vegetable oils. Polyunsaturated and monounsaturated fats are found in vegetable oils, nuts, seeds, and fish. They lower disease risks. Stay away from saturated fats found in red meats and full-fat dairy and from trans fats, hydrogenated oils, found in processed foods and baked goods. However, our bodies absolutely need good fats to function well.

- Use whole grains as a good source of fiber and important nutrients such as selenium, magnesium, and potassium.

- Use low-fat proteins, such as skinless chicken breast, beans, and nuts, and lean cuts of beef and pork. And have two servings a week of fish.

- Keep your salt intake to about 1 teaspoon a day (2400 mg. sodium). Make it ½ teaspoon a day (1200 mg. sodium) for seniors and others who need to limit their salt intake. Most of your salt intake comes from the processed, packaged, and fast-foods. Using a salt-shaker limits your use of salt.

- Limit sugars to about 10 teaspoons a day (40 g).

As you can see, it's very simple.

The difficulty is in changing our typical American eating habits, and they are habits, to meet these simple guidelines. We have learned to eat the way we do now over a period of years.

We can also learn to eat in a new way so that we have much more energy and so that we can begin to conquer obesity and the many health-related diseases that plague us. Not only will we feel good; we'll also feel good about ourselves.

Plan to Eat Right

Planning includes deciding what to buy, where to get the food, how much food is needed, and determining portion sizes. It is planning to be healthy and alert because of the choices you make.

Not only will we feel good; we'll also feel good about ourselves.

Start slowly and mindfully as you take action. Be aware. Eating well is an important first step. Adding exercise and getting enough rest to relieve stress will complete the task. A healthy life with all its benefits is then yours.

This book makes beginning and sticking with healthy eating easy because the healthy eating plan includes menus and amazingly easy recipes and shortcuts. And, importantly, *this is not a gourmet cookbook*. These are delicious recipes that are easy and simple to make so that anyone can be healthy. There are many shortcuts included, and still the recipes are healthy.

So come on! Let's go. The food is delicious. Cooking it is actually easy. And, most importantly, you'll feel good.

About the Menus and Recipes

The menus are geared to the seasons—the hot and the cold. They all provide a healthy balanced diet. Recipes follow each menu, and they're simple, making this an easy meal plan to follow. Notes on many of the ingredients chosen for a healthy diet are included after the first mention of the ingredient.

In addition, Chapter 15, "Celebrations!," pages 187-223, contains menus and recipes that are simple to prepare yet fancy in appearance. They will serve for holidays, birthdays, anniversaries, or any other special occasions.

Additional recipes are included in Chapter 16, "More Healthy, Easy Recipes," pages 224-253, and most of the recipes there are recommended as substitutes to the recipes in a day's menu.

Sidestepping the Recommended Menus and Recipes

Face it. There are many times we simply don't have the time to sit down to eat, much less shop for the ingredients in a recipe and then cook it. Sidestepping this critical piece of a healthy lifestyle won't benefit you as much as taking the time to embrace a full and healthy eating practice. You can, though, incorporate the rules for healthy eating into your grab-and-go meals.

Breakfast is the foundation for a healthy lifestyle and healthy eating.

Yet, most of us are rushed, especially for breakfast. That's when you want to be sure to include a good serving of protein with whole grains and vegetables or fruit—but to avoid bad fats, high sugar, and white flour.

Protein, whenever you eat it, gives you sustenance and satisfaction for hours and lasts till you have your next meal. The good carbohydrates found in fruits and vegetables give you the energy you need to be your best.

Even when you're rushed, you can still consume a healthy diet. For example, for breakfast on-the-go, you could

- Grab a slice of reduced fat cheese and wrap it in a slice of whole grain bread. Then take a banana or apple to eat with it and a bottle of plain water.

- Or for lunch take a peeled, hard-boiled egg and add whole grain crackers and fruit or a vegetable along with a bottle of water.

See how simple that is? You've got yourself quick, healthy, balanced meals.

There are other options, of course. You can get up out of bed 15 minutes earlier than usual. Just 15 minutes. That way you'll have time to fix eggs or oatmeal and prepare a lunch of leftovers from previous meals.

The reality, though, is that most of us will be unable to cook every meal for one reason or another. When that happens, keep the rule of three in your planning—include:

- vegetables and fruit,

- whole grain, and

- protein in each meal.

Good luck!

You Can Succeed!

Begin this new way of eating gradually so that you are more likely to succeed.

- Gradually cut down on the amount of salt, sugar, saturated fats, and simple carbohydrates that are based on white flour and sugar.

- Gradually substitute a healthy way of eating in a lifestyle that also involves exercise and adequate rest.

- Give yourself a chance to succeed, and you will find yourself full of energy, stamina, and positive feelings about yourself. (See Chapter 5, "Tips: Making Healthy Eating Easier," pages 23-27, for ideas that will help you succeed.)

Plan to Make Healthy Eating a Vital Part of Your Life

If you find yourself straying from the healthy eating plan, go back to it the next day or even the next meal. There's nothing wrong with eating a piece of your birthday cake. However, it leads you far away from your healthy diet if you find yourself eating the whole thing. There's nothing wrong with occasionally grabbing a quick bite at a fast food outlet. Just don't get the fries and soda to go with it.

Be sure to include daily exercise and adequate rest in your life along with healthy eating. Exercise, rest, and healthy eating are the basis of a long and healthy life.

You can do it!

Chapter 5

Tips

Making Healthy Eating Easier

Number one tip?

Don't try to make the changes all at once. Start slowly, but not too slowly! Add more fruits and vegetables, whole grains, and lean proteins to your diet gradually. You can build on your choices. You are trading your old, unhealthy habits for new, healthy ones. Your plan is to avoid the diseases that accompany an unhealthy lifestyle.

Use these simple strategies to become healthy:

- Always, always read the Nutrition Facts label, located on the back of a food package. It's your friend and will help you make the right choices for your diet. There is a complete discussion of this label in Chapter 9, "Nutrition Facts Labels: What They Are Really Saying," pages 56-58. An even better way to eating healthy is to avoid foods that have to carry a Nutrition Facts label. Having no label means those foods are fresh and haven't been processed by a manufacturer.

- Don't skip meals, especially not breakfast. If you do, you'll feel sluggish and make poor eating choices later in the day. This is not deprivation diet. If you allow yourself to become starved, you'll eat much more to satisfy both the emotional and physical needs that have built up.

- But serving size is important. Keep the amount you eat to a reasonable size. Check the Nutrition Facts label for what the manufacturer considers a serving. (What the manufacturer considers a serving often isn't related to reality!)

- According to the USDA 2012 guidelines, My Plate, each meal divides one plate into three sections based on calories—30 percent whole grains, 50 percent vegetables and fruits, and 20 percent protein. This ideal plate is accompanied by dairy, such as low-fat or skim milk or yogurt. You might choose another kind of "milk." (See page 41 for kinds of "milk." If you choose another "milk," check its nutritional value on the Nutrition Facts label on the backs of the product.)

- Serving sizes make a difference. You can use the following as your guide:

  - Proteins: A serving of meat is about 2 to 3 ounces, or the size of a deck of cards. Other protein serving sizes: 2 to 3 tablespoons nut butters, 2 to 3 eggs, and ½ cup dry beans before they are cooked and 1 to 1½ cups cooked.

  - Whole grains: A serving is 1 slice whole grain bread, ½ cup of prepared cereal, or ½ cup of cooked pasta or rice.

  - Fruit or vegetables: A serving is ½ cup chopped fruit or vegetable. You need 4 to 6 servings per day.

  - Dairy: A serving equals the following dairy products: 1 cup milk or yogurt, low-fat or skim; ½ to 1 cup cottage cheese, low-fat or fat-free; or 1 ounce cheese, reduced-fat or low-fat. Approximate serving sizes for other kinds of "milk" is about the same. Check the Nutrition Facts label.

- Don't count calories but watch your portion sizes. This is not a deprivation diet. Know approximately how many calories and what size portion you need to maintain or lose weight.

See Chapter 9, "Nutrition Facts Labels: What They Are Really Saying," pages 56-58.

- As we have emphasized, breakfast is the most important meal of the day. A good breakfast with protein, fruit, and whole grains will give you energy and a satisfied feeling that will last for hours.

- Healthy snacks will keep your body energized and full, so you won't gorge later because you're famished. Good carbohydrates energize you and protein fills you. Eat all your between-meals scheduled snacks that are in your menus, but be sure they are healthy snacks, not sugared or salted junk food. Each day's menus have recommendations for healthy snacks, and you can read about snacking in Chapter 10, "Munching! Snacks for a Healthy Diet," pages 59-62.

- Nuts and seeds are essential to a healthy diet, but you must be aware that many packages of nuts and seeds are highly salted. Look for unsalted, raw nuts that are usually available in the produce section of the grocery store.

  - You'll find directions for roasting raw nuts and seeds with each recipe and in Chapter 16, "More Healthy, Easy Recipes," page 224. There's also information on nuts and seeds in Chapter 8, "Healthy Eating Nutrition: Briefly," pages 49.

  - Watch your portion sizes. Usually two 1-ounce servings a day of nuts and seeds won't add to your weight gain and will give you the nutrients you need.

- Low-fat and reduced-fat cheeses are a good source of protein and calcium. However, choose lower fat cheeses or use a minimum amount of any cheese such as one slice or a few sprinkles of shredded cheese. Naturally low-fat cheeses are part-skim mozzarella, string cheeses, farmer's cheese, Neufchatel (low-fat cream cheese), and goat cheese. Low-fat and reduced-fat cheeses can be found in cheddar, Monterey Jack, mozzarella, Brie, Swiss, Colby, Muenster, and American. Read the Nutrition Facts labels found on cheese packages.

- When you want something sweet, first choose fruit such as a banana, grapes, or an orange. That'll usually satisfy your craving. Realize that you're going to feel cravings for the junk food that you ate in the past. Expect it.

- Vegetables and fruits should be the staples of your diet. Cook and serve them as simply as possible, avoiding heavy sauces or toppings. You can serve and eat many of them steamed or raw.

You're going to feel cravings for the junk food that you ate in the past. Expect it.

- Find healthy substitutes. When you get the urge to eat unhealthy foods, take a walk outside, call a friend, or do something else rewarding. Soon you'll find junk food won't satisfy you, but fruits and vegetables—whether fresh, dried, canned, or frozen—will.

- Stay away from white flour as much as possible. Buy whole wheat and whole grain pasta, breads, and baked goods. Use whole grains in your recipes that you make at home, such as wheat, rye, oat, or spelt. See the section on whole grains in Chapter 8, "Healthy Eating Nutrition: Briefly," page 49.

- No caffeine after noon. Coffee, most teas, and chocolate all contain caffeine. However, there are many herb and decaffeinated teas available.

- Buy fruits and vegetables in season when you can. They taste brighter when they are fresh. Freezing and canning uses fruits and vegetables right after they've been picked in the fields, so their nutrition levels are excellent. If you buy prepared fruits and vegetables, avoid any with added salt and sugar.

- If you have trouble sleeping on a full stomach or if you have acid reflux, eat your nighttime meal two or three hours before you go to bed. Your body needs time to slow down for a good night's sleep. Many people eat their biggest meal at a much earlier hour, such as lunchtime.

- Have desserts only with your main meal. Often it is dinner but sometimes lunch.

- Nutritionists say that three to four smaller meals during the day is the best way to eat.

- Alcohol adds calories to your daily nutrients and not much else.

IF YOU LIKE TO BAKE

You can make your recipes healthier by substituting for saturated fats and high-calorie oils. If you replace the fat in baked goods with substitutes, the baking time is usually shorter. Begin checking for doneness 10 minutes before the recipe's time is up.

- Fruit purees: Applesauce, mashed bananas, pureed peaches and pears, and prune puree are examples of fruit puree substitutes. Use about half as much of the fruit puree as the total amount of fat called for in the recipe. You can add more puree if the mixture looks dry.

- Vegetable purees can also be used. For example, mashed squashes (like pumpkin) or sweet potatoes are used. You can use ¾ as much of the vegetable puree as the total amount of fat called for in the recipe. Add more puree if the batter looks dry.

- Fat-free yogurt or buttermilk works as fat substitutes. Use ¾ of the substitute for the fat called for in the recipe, adding more if the mixture is dry.

Chapter 6

Stock Your Kitchen

With Healthy, Delicious Food

"Your food shall be your medicine and your medicine shall be your food."
Hippocrates, Greek physician and philosopher

Cleaning Out and Stocking Up

Cleaning out won't be done without a lot of teeth gnashing. You're throwing away food you love and have paid for. But it's the first real step to gaining, or regaining, your health.

If you truly believe that you won't binge on these foods, then keep some handy. Realistically, most of us won't be able to resist the lure of these foods. Then you need to clean out your kitchen. Your health comes before satisfaction.

When you clean out, first get rid of all your temptations, of all your bad stuff. It won't be easy, but by doing so you'll ensure that your new lifestyle has a chance of succeeding.

Go through your cabinets and remove cake mix boxes, cookies, bags of chips and candy, coupons to fast food restaurants, donuts, large bagels, energy bars that are really candy bars, both diet and sugared soft drinks, pizza, and all the other hidden, unhealthy foods that are calling you.

You'll go through your refrigerator and freezer and remove your bacon, lunch meats, jams and jellies with high fructose corn syrup, blocks of high-fat cheeses, whole milk and products made of whole milk, ice cream, sherbet, frozen chicken wings and other processed snacks and dinners, and all the food that does not add to your good health.

You know what should go, don't you? That task shouldn't take long.

The difficult part is throwing away old habits. But you can do it because you've made the decision to be healthy.

Now you're ready to restock your pantry with foods you'll use often in your new healthy eating plan. Now you'll be ready to put together a quick meal without having to run to the store every time you cook. Now you're ready to become vital, strong, and full of verve.

The basic shopping list below includes foods that are smart to have available in your healthy kitchen. It's the basis of the new healthy eating plan that's for you.

Basic Shopping List for Easy Cooking and a Healthy Kitchen

- Cans of diced tomatoes, salt-free if available

- Cans of tomato sauce, salt-free if available

- Cans of whole tomatoes, salt-free if available

- Packages of dried beans, 16-ounces, any kind

- Cans of cooked beans, any kind

- Dried fruits, any kind

- Milk and milk products, low-fat or skim, including plain yogurt, Greek yogurt, string cheese, cottage cheese, or "milk" of your choice. (See page 41 for kinds of "milk.")

- Eggs

- Extra virgin olive oil

- Canola oil

- Vinegar, any kind such as Balsamic, apple cider, white, or your choice

- Whole wheat flour: Milling the white wheat produces a light-textured whole wheat. The brown flour that most of us associate with whole wheat is milled from red wheat.

- Whole grain flour: Any kind of whole grain, including soy, oat, spelt, rye, and many more kinds.

- Breads, crackers, whole grain baked goods, including tortillas, pita, and Nabisco Graham Crackers, or other graham cracker without added high fructose corn syrup.

- Whole grain cereal, such as Cheerios, Skinner's Raisin Bran, All Bran, Wheaties, and so forth, with no added sugar, fat, or salt.

- Hot cereals, such as oatmeal, old fashioned, quick, or instant with no added sugars or fats; Ralston; Wheatena; and so forth, with no added sugar, fat, or salt.

- Nuts, unsalted, including almonds and walnuts

- Nut butters, natural with no added salt, sugar, or fat

- Hummus, prepared or homemade

- Honey

- Jams, preserves, and jellies, all natural fruit spread without added sugar, if possible, or sweetened with fruit juice

- Lettuce, fresh fruits, and vegetables, especially colorful produce and dark lettuce

- Canned and frozen fruits and veggies, without added salt or sugar. Frozen contains the most nutrients because it is frozen immediately after harvest.

- Dried or fresh herbs and spices of various kinds (see below)

- Garlic, fresh, powdered, or dried

- Onion, fresh or dried

- Whole grain sides, such as rice, brown; whole wheat couscous and other whole wheat pastas; barley; bulgur; quinoa; wild rice; and many other kinds of whole grains

Warning: Coupons in the newspaper, online, or in magazines are for high-priced, overly processed, high-sugar, high-fat, high-salt foods. You don't save money by using them and they lead you to sabotage your diet. Buy store brands and foods that aren't so highly processed instead. That way you actually save money and your health.

Kick Up the Taste

Some Common Herbs and Spices

This list of herbs and spices is useful when you need guidance in picking out your own flavorings. There are recommendations in each recipe. However, be adventurous. Try herbs and spices that are new for you. Buy the ones on sale or fresh in the market. Most dishes will taste just as good when you select the herbs and spices that you'd prefer, even if they weren't in the recipe.

When you're using herbs, usually, it's best to put fresh herbs in a cooking dish close to the time it will finish cooking. That's true for dried herbs as well, though you can put them in as you sauté the basic vegetables before adding sauces. The ratio of fresh to dried herbs is usually one tablespoon of fresh herbs to one teaspoon dried. You can keep fresh herbs longer by placing the cut ends in a glass of water. Keep the dried herbs in a cool, dark place, or even in the freezer.

Finally, enjoy what you're cooking! The aromas that drift to you from the added herbs and spices actually enhance the flavor and greatly increase your enjoyment of the dish.

The recipes in this book use herbs and spices to kick up the taste without adding extra salt and sugar. A listing of the herbs and spices you'll most often find in these recipes or elsewhere are:

Herbs

Basil: This herb grows fast in the summer. There's a sweet fragrance to it, dried or fresh, and it goes well with tomato dishes, soups, stews, eggs, and salads. Keep at least a container of dried basil on hand. When you can get fresh, store it with the cut end in a glass of water, as with most fresh herbs.

Bay Leaves: These leaves are from the bay laurel tree and are used whole in soups, stews, and other dishes. After cooking, the leaves are removed from the dish before serving. The leaves only develop their full flavor several weeks after they are picked and dried.

Cilantro or Coriander: Some call it cilantro; others call it coriander, or even Chinese parsley. It adds zest to any Mexican-style dish such as chili and you can use it to beef up salsas, soups, stews, curries, salads, vegetables, fish, and chicken dishes or just about any food you love. A big bunch of fresh cilantro costs less than a dollar. Some people do not like cilantro.

Dill: Fresh dill has feathery leaves and it goes well with fish, potato salad, cucumbers, and even pickles. Like most herbs, you can use it wherever you wish.

Oregano: This perennial herb grows almost wildly either in pots or in the ground. Use oregano in scrambled eggs, quiche, pizza, tomato sauce, salad dressing, and on chicken or seafood. Put fresh oregano in a glass of water, and you'll see roots grow. Keep a container of dried oregano on hand and fresh whenever you happen to find it. Marjoram is often substituted for oregano and is sweeter with a more delicate taste.

Parsley: Keep a bunch of parsley in the refrigerator or a container of dried parsley nearby for use in most of your dishes. It's mild and has a slightly grassy flavor that goes very well with salads. Flat-leaf parsley is the kind we usually use in cooking while curly parsley is more decorative. You can use curly parsley for celebrations or special dinners.

Rosemary: This herb is a woody shrub and the cuttings root easily. The leaves are needle-like with a pine and lemony flavor. It goes well with lamb, pizza, tomato sauce, and garlic. However, it's strong so use it sparingly.

Sage: Sage, like most of the herbs, is native to the Mediterranean. It has long, narrow, gray-green leaves and goes well with soups, stews, turkey dressing, pork, and many other dishes. Use it sparingly as its strength can dominate a dish.

Tarragon: This herb is not native to the Mediterranean but is from Siberia and western Asia. The French use it widely and its sweet, delicate flavor and perfume go well with fish, omelets, chicken, and sauces. You can grow it as a perennial. Keep a container of dried tarragon on hand and buy fresh when you can find it. Because of its distinctive flavor, a little goes a long way.

Thyme: This herb is a perennial, woody shrub and has small leaves growing on long stems. It is an ancient plant used by Egyptians and Greeks. Thyme, related to mint, can be used with eggs, soups, stews, beans, and many other dishes. You can use dried, the leaves, or the whole stems that you remove when the dish is cooked. Keep a container of dried thyme on hand.

Spices

Allspice: This is usually found as a ground powder and can be substituted for cloves. Use it in pumpkin recipes, baked goods, and stews.

Cloves: This spice is from the flower bud of a tree grown in India, Pakistan, and throughout the Southeast Asia area. In its ground form, it is often used in desserts as well as in savory dishes. It is used whole with ham and other meats. Cloves also have medicinal uses as they have a numbing effect on mouth tissues.

Chili Powder: This spice comes from the dried, pulverized chili peppers and is used in a number of dishes to add heat and spice to dishes such as chili. It can be hot or mild.

Cinnamon: This spice is found either as sticks, when it is placed whole in dishes as they cook and removed before serving, or as ground, when it is added to any number of sweet or savory dishes. Cinnamon is from the tree's inner bark and is native to Southeast Asia.

Cumin: This spice grows as an annual plant in the Mediterranean area. Though cooks in the United States usually find it ground, it is used either ground or whole in cuisines all over the world, especially Middle Eastern, Asian, Mediterranean, and Mexican cuisines. The easiest way to use it is ground and it goes well with beans, chili, and soups. Cumin is one of the main ingredients in curry powder. The Cubans use it frequently in their cuisine. Keep a container on hand.

Curry: Curry powder is actually a mixture of spices. It usually is a blend of coriander, turmeric, cumin, fenugreek, and red pepper with additions of other spices depending on the cook and creator. Curry is used in Indian cuisine, and it can be added to several other dishes such as bean soups, including lentil and dried green pea for a kick.

Ginger: Ginger comes from the rhizome (root) of the flowering subtropical plant often found in gardens or used in flower arrangements. It can be used powdered in desserts, such as pumpkin pie, ginger bread, and the like, and it is found in ginger ale, ginger tea, and ginger wine. It is used in many curry dishes, stews, and soups. It can be candied and is found as crystallized ginger. Japanese, Chinese, and Koreans often pickle fresh ginger slices.

Nutmeg: This spice grows on trees found in Indonesia as well as in the Caribbean. Usually used in its ground form, nutmeg, and its red, lacy covering known as mace, can be found in sweet as well as savory dishes. It perks up many dishes such as beans, soups, cakes, and pumpkin dishes. Keep either the whole nutmeg or ground nutmeg on hand.

Paprika: This spice is ground from the dried fruits of either bell pepper or a chili pepper. Paprika is often used to season and color rice, stews, and soups. Its effects range from hot to mild. You can sprinkle it on foods as a garnish.

Saving Money and Shopping Healthy

You can do both—have healthy meals and save money. Some tips for frugal, healthy shopping follow:

Protein Sources

Meat: Eat red meat only occasionally. Unfortunately, lean and extra-lean varieties tend to be more expensive than fatter cuts. Filet mignon, which has a lot of saturated marbled fat, is probably not going to be on your menu, but extra-lean or lean ground beef might be. In this case, consider buying larger, fresh packs, so the unit cost of the meat is lower. Use what you need for your planned meal, and then freeze the rest in serving size containers or zip lock bags.

Plus, if a recipe calls for a pound of lean ground beef, consider using only ½ to ¾ of a pound instead and adding ground turkey, chicken, mashed beans, or oatmeal or other whole grains. Your meat will stretch further, and you'll reduce the amount of fat in your meals.

Lean cuts of meat like beef round steak tend to be tough cuts. These cook beautifully in a slow cooker or by braising slowly in a large skillet, so you can still enjoy relatively inexpensive, fork-tender meat.

Again, use meat sparingly, making up only 20 percent of your daily calories, so that it accents your meal rather than dominates it.

Poultry: Boneless, skinless chicken breasts can be very expensive. These would be good items to buy in larger quantities if you have space. The unit cost of buying chicken in a larger package will be less than choosing a package with just two chicken breasts or selecting them piece by piece from the meat counter.

When you buy larger packages of chicken breast, pack them for the freezer carefully. Prepare serving sizes of the raw breasts by placing wax paper or plastic wrap between each breast and putting them in a freezer zip-lock bag. You can store these wrapped, raw breasts for up to nine months.

Buy plain chicken breasts rather than pre-seasoned or marinated chicken, both of which contain salt and fats.

Chicken thighs are cheaper than chicken breasts, and so long as you remove the skin or buy already skinless thighs, you won't consume a significant amount of extra fat. Thigh meat is rich and flavorful, so you don't need much of it.

Occasionally, you will find that a whole chicken is cheaper than buying packs of chicken breasts. Roast the chicken and remove the skin and fat before eating it. Use leftovers in soups or sandwiches.

Fish: Fish can be expensive, so see if there are any good deals on fresh varieties. Tilapia and sole are relatively cheap. If the cost is prohibitive, choose frozen fish fillets or fish steaks. Opt for plain fillets rather than breaded or marinated fish. Plain fillets are lower in fat, sodium, and other additives. If fresh fish happens to be on sale, buy some for today and some for your freezer.

Beans: Beans are a cheap and wonderful alternative source of protein. Canned beans may seem reasonably cheap, but you can get a lot more for your money if you buy dried beans and cook them yourself. It's easy. (See the recipe for cooking dried beans, page 225.) Plus, canned beans are usually high in sodium though they are exceptionally convenient and can be healthy if you rinse them well before using.

Dairy: If money is tight, then you won't want to pay extra for organic low-fat milk. Buy what you can afford for drinking and consider buying instant milk powder, which has become a delicious alternative to fresh milk. You can use buttermilk powder for baking. Low-fat or skim milk should be no more expensive than whole milk.

A fat-free half-and-half cream is available and is a tasty addition to your coffee or tea, and works well with cut-up fruit. It doesn't have a lot of nutritional value and isn't low in calories, so keep that in mind when you plan to use it.

Buy blocks of reduced-fat cheese and grate it yourself rather than buying packs of pre-shredded cheese. Again, reduced-fat cheese shouldn't be more expensive than regular cheese.

Buy stronger flavor cheeses over milder ones and use smaller amounts. You'll get the flavor for fewer calories, and your cheese supply will last longer. Pre-sliced cheese is more expensive than blocks. Slice your own! Pre-sliced, though, is a great convenience for a busy person.

Light ice cream or frozen yogurt shouldn't be more expensive than regular ice cream and should still be an occasional treat, not an everyday dessert. If you buy a large container, enjoy it only once a week. Stick to a half-cup serving size, and the tub will stretch further!

Fruits and Vegetables

Yes, fresh produce can be expensive, but if you're cutting back on processed snacks and non-essential packaged foods, you can afford some fresh fruit and veggies. Snacking on carrots, bell peppers, and broccoli rather than salty fat-filled crackers and chips is so much better for you. Fresh produce will last much longer than you might expect.

The same goes for fruit. Pre-cut cantaloupe or pineapple is much more expensive than buying the whole fruit. Plus, some of the vitamins may be lost if the cut items have been sitting around for a while.

Buy in season. Asparagus in November is going to be expensive, but much less so in April and May. Cherries in February are not even worth considering, but much more affordable in June. Packaged salad mixes and bagged pre-washed lettuce are more expensive than a head of lettuce, but they are a convenience. If having packaged mixes makes a difference in how you eat, then use them by all means.

Packaged salad mixes and bagged pre-washed lettuces are more expensive than a head of lettuce, but they are a convenience.

When it comes to apples and oranges, it actually does pay to buy the bagged version rather than the loose variety. However, one apple or orange will last a long time, even if cut, placed in a container, and refrigerated.

Frozen fruit and vegetables can be economical and there is more vitamin and mineral content in frozen foods than in fresh because they have been frozen or canned when immediately harvested. When there's a sale, stock up on as many frozen fruits and vegetables as you can. Be sure there is no added sugar, salt, or fat in these products.

Consider growing your own veggies and herbs in pots or a garden patch. It may not be less expensive, but it's a delight to pick a few leaves of your own herbs to put into your cooked meals or salads.

Canned and Packaged Goods
Store brands are cheaper than name brands, from pasta to cereal to beans, vegetables and fruit to tuna fish. These are just as nutritious as nationally known brands that spend a lot on advertising.

Choose low-sodium canned goods, water-packed meat or tuna, and water-packed or low-sugar canned fruit. Canned tomatoes are a great bargain, as they can be used in so many recipes. Look for low sodium (salt). Buy whole-grain rice and pasta in large packages instead of small boxes, and store them in the refrigerator because they may turn rancid at room temperatures.

Freezing What You Cook
You can cook more than a recipe calls for and freeze the remainder in serving-size containers for future use. That's an energy saver.

Condiments
These items tend to be occasional purchases, so you can buy smaller sizes and they will last a long time. Use sparingly. They are usually high in sodium (salt), sugar, and/or fat.

Beverages
Do you really need bottled water? Probably not. Tap water is safe and is cheap. (See the Chapter 7, "Drink Up! What You Drink is Important," pp. 40-44.) Skip the soda and sugary juice drinks because they add calories rather than good nutrients. Spend your money on drinks like milk that will add to your health. If you want something refreshing, try some of the herb teas.

Coupon Smarts

Face it. Most coupons are for expensive, highly processed foods that are high in fat, salt, and sugar. Don't fall for them. You can save a lot more money and stay healthy by buying store brands and healthy foods that are on sale. You'll do yourself a favor if you don't cut coupons!

Saving Package Leftovers

Most of the time you won't use everything in a package that you buy. Carefully save what is left by putting a rubber band around the opened package, closing it with a clothespin, taping it with masking tape, pouring what is left in a plastic container or baggie, and putting these leftovers in the pantry or refrigerator for future use. Place leftover canned or frozen goods in containers and refrigerate or freeze until you use them.

Chapter 7

Drink Up!

What You Drink Is Important

Beverages in the Plan

Did you know that a major portion of your daily intake is of liquid? That's vital, of course, since about two-thirds of our bodies is water. How you get that water into your body makes a huge difference in your health, in whether you gain pounds through empty calories, adding sugar that leads to illness and weight gain.

When you want something to drink, think of plain water first. Water keeps our bodies working. It's cheap and, coming out of the tap, it's safe. And it doesn't add calories and sugar like sodas or juices or even sweetened coffee or tea.

Drinks Good for You

Water

Your cells and body are mostly water. You'll never go wrong if you choose to drink water, and lots of it. A study published by the journal *Nephrology* and conducted by researchers at the University of Sydney in Australia showed that those who drank the most water had significantly lower chronic kidney disease.

There's an urban myth that you should drink eight glasses of water a day. That's not proved by research. Even so, be sure to drink enough water so that your urine is light, not dark yellow. And increase the amount of water you drink year by year as you grow older. You'll need more water then to keep your body working right.

The best water is what you drink water right out of the tap. You can cool it in the refrigerator in the summer. Tap water has been purified by your city's water purification plant. (If you use well water, have it tested for contaminants.)

If you prefer filtered water because of the taste, you can put a filter on the tap so that each glass is immediately filtered. Or you can filter a pitcher at a time. (A whole house filter is usually reverse osmosis and is costly.) As far as so-called filtered bottled water is concerned, most brands are really just tap water.

Very few brands of commercial bottled water list the sources of their water to show that their water is not tap water. The three brands that list the sources of their water as well as the methods they use to purify the water are: Gerber Purified Water, Nestle Pure Life Purified Water, and Penta Ultra-Purified Water.

Lots of people like flavored water, no matter from where they get it. You can flavor your water yourself, saving money and assuring that you know what's in your water. Try adding a sliver of lime or lemon to a pitcher or glass of water. Or you can put in another type of fruit or vegetable cut into pieces or sliced. I've had cucumber slices in a cold pitcher of water, for example. You could put in strawberries, pineapple pieces, or other favorites. Experiment.

Herb teas count as water. These teas are flavored with mint, chamomile, or a number of other healthful herbs and, like most teas, are very refreshing and soothing. Avoid teas made with licorice, ephedra, or comfrey, each of which has been linked to health problems.

Milk and "Milk"

Milk is almost a miracle food. It has antibodies, protein, calcium, fat, and many other essential nutrients. Most of us drink milk from female cows, and newborn humans and infants nurse from their mothers because mammal milk has all those nutrients.

Trouble is that whole milk also contains high amounts of saturated fats, which is good for infants, but not so good for adults.

That's why low-fat or skim milk is popular and most often used in healthy diets.

Buy pasteurized skim or low-fat milk because pasteurizing kills disease-causing organisms. Homogenizing milk is a mechanical process that allows producers to remove separated fat molecules to make low-fat and skim milk.

Some prefer other kinds of "milk" such as soy, goat, rice, almond, sheep, hemp, oat, coconut, flax seed, and others. These other kinds of "milk" may not give you the nutrients you want, instead giving you empty calories. Please check the Nutrition Facts label on each "milk" carton or can.

Drinks Good in Moderation

Coffee

It used to be thought that coffee was bad for you. Now there are studies that show it is good for you. Why? Because caffeine contains most of our needed daily intake of antioxidants that destroy free radicals. (This is true for not only coffee with caffeine but also decaf.)

What are free radicals? These are unstable molecules in our bodies that aren't all bad. For example, they help white blood cells attack bacteria and pathogens. They cause damage, though, when they damage our healthy molecules and then speed up our aging processes. There are several diseases linked to free radicals that destroy our healthy molecules: Alzheimer's, Type 2 diabetes, heart disease, and Parkinson's disease; in women they are linked to stroke.

That's a simple explanation of why coffee is good for you.

Regular coffee, of course, has its problem. Since it contains caffeine, it raises blood pressure and the levels of adrenaline in the blood. Watch how much you drink every day. Usually two cups is considered a safe amount.

Don't add much sugar or cream to your cup of coffee because when you do you're adding empty calories and cholesterol. If you do put these into your coffee, keep them to a minimum. A popular substitute for regular half-and-half cream is the fat-free half-and-half that's also delicious on fruits and cereals, and in soups, and other items that seem to cry out for cream.

Tea

Tea is one of the most satisfying drinks, either hot or cold. It is soothing, calming, and, in the heat of the summer, cooling. However, be sure to order or buy your tea unsweetened. Add sugar or honey yourself. That way you're in control of how much sweetener you consume. Commercially sweetened tea has much too much sugar, both sucrose, or table sugar, and high fructose corn syrup. Any sugar in excess is bad for you and your liver.

You can make your own sugar syrup that will blend into cold tea more easily than table sugar by mixing a half cup of sugar with one cup of water, stir over heat until the sugar dissolves, and place the sugar-water mixture in a jar. Add a scant spoonful to your iced tea as needed, always using as little as possible.

The need for sweetened tea is really a habit you've learned, and it's not a good habit. An unsweetened cup of hot tea or tall glass of iced tea can be just as satisfying as sweetened tea. You can start out with unsweetened green tea and herbal teas that don't need much sugar. When I add milk to my hot tea, I don't need any sugar.

Drinks Not Good

Juice

We have been told that fruit juice is good for us. Yet fruit juice is actually high in sugar content and has little or no fiber. Whole fruits, with all their micro- and macronutrients are far better for you than juice. Keep your juice drinking to a minimum and turn to water, low-fat or skim milk, or unsweetened tea instead.

Drinks to Avoid

Sodas

Loaded with sugars and carbonation, sodas are not good for you. The sugars alone add empty calories to your diet. Plus, studies show that carbonation in sodas leaches calcium from our bones. It also causes acid reflux that could lead to cancer of the esophagus.

We've already indicated that large amounts of sugars can lead to diabetes and other major illnesses. And don't try to fix the problem by drinking diet sodas. Those artificial sweeteners hook you into craving overly sweet foods.

If you like fizzy drinks, try buying plain sparkling water and adding a piece of fruit such as a slice of apple, a strawberry, or lemon peel, same as you would add to flavor your water.

Alcohol

Alcohol, especially red wine, has heart-healthy resveratrol, an anti-inflammatory found in many plants as well. With that information alone, you'd think that alcohol itself is good for the health and your heart. But that's true only if you consume very little alcohol, keeping your total consumption to one or two drinks a day.

If you don't drink alcohol, don't start now because you think it's good for you.

You can get the same or better benefits from red and purple grape juices, dark chocolate, cranberries, blueberries, pomegranates, and peanuts.

Drink Enough

Try to drink enough to keep your body working its best and drink only those liquids that don't destroy your good intentions. That means drink as much plain water as you can, lots of low-fat or skim milk, "milk" of your choice, some coffee, and unsweetened teas. Skip sodas, juices, and alcohol. You don't really need those empty calories at all.

Chapter 8

Healthy Eating Nutrition

Briefly

Passport to a Long, Healthy Life

You're on the way to a long and healthy life when you adopt the simple and easy healthy eating plan described on pages 68-71. Heart disease caused by too much bad fat that clogs arteries, diabetes caused by too much sugar and too little exercise, high blood pressure caused by too much salt—these diseases are much more likely to be avoided if you eat healthily.

When you follow this healthy eating plan, the great variety of foods you enjoy will supply most of your needed nutrients. You might need a good multivitamin as insurance, but most of you won't need a closet full of vitamin and mineral supplements. That's a money and time saver, but be sure to talk with your doctor about your specific needs.

It's important to know that a healthy diet includes a balance of several nutrients. You absolutely need the good kinds of fat, a variety of fruits and vegetables, lean proteins of many kinds, and whole grains. And you must keep added salt and sugar to a minimum

The details of this essential and healthy diet are as follows:

Vegetables and Fruits

Colorful fruits and vegetables are the foundation of healthy eating. Choose orange, red, purple, green, and yellow; and plan your menu around them. Fresh, canned, or frozen fruits and vegetables are excellent, and all will be chock full of nutrients and micronutrients.

A busy person often has to buy canned, frozen, or prepared fruits and vegetables, or dried herbs. Their foods won't be gourmet but they'll be both healthy and delicious.

Whenever you can, buy fresh because preparing them for cooking or adding to salads is simple and not at all time consuming. When you buy fresh, you probably buy the fruits and vegetables when they are in season and the flavors are at their peak. When buying canned and some frozen, you will see they often have added salt, possibly sugar, and sometimes fat. Check the Nutrition Facts labels on the backs of these products.

Vegetables and fruits are a good source of fiber, the major nutrients, and multiple micronutrients, all necessary for the top functioning of our bodies and minds. A study in the *American Journal of Clinical Nutrition* has shown that people who ate the most fruits and vegetables had the highest scores on verbal tests. In other words, fruits and vegetables contribute to a better memory.

Leafy greens, especially, provide us with many necessary nutrients. That's why you'll usually find a salad in most of the menus in this book and a recommendation that you keep leafy salad greens in your refrigerator.

And if you find you simply don't have the time or energy to wash and tear lettuce for a salad, buy and keep the packaged, pre-washed lettuces on hand.

Eating as many as five to ten servings a day of vegetables and fruits may be new to you. Start slowly. Adjust by adding a portion at a time. Soon you'll find your plate is three-quarters full of vegetables and fruits. And you might even find that you prefer it that way.

Proteins

According to studies completed at George Washington University, proteins are central to maintaining a healthy body, they help repair cells and build new ones, and they regulate many of the body's actions. Proteins are vital to breaking down the nutrients you consume into usable components. And proteins are linked to the production of energy and stamina. The Mayo Clinic states that protein is essential for growth and development, and all the cells of your body include protein.

There are so many available sources of protein, both plant and animal based, that it's easy to get too much. Only 10 to 35 percent of your calories should be from protein.

Though you may try to avoid the saturated fats found in some meats and full-fat dairy products, there are still many types of lean proteins. These include eggs and egg whites; low-fat and fat-free dairy products; dried beans; nuts and seeds; lean cuts of beef, lamb, pork, white meat chicken and poultry without the skin; and, of course, fish.

Meats, if lean, are high-quality protein and have little saturated fats. You can make a hamburger or meatloaf with part chopped 93% to 96% lean beef combined with other kinds of chopped lean meats such as chicken, turkey, and pork loin; oatmeal or other whole grains; and cooked dried beans, any kind. Black beans not only taste especially good with ground meat, they also blend in with the cooked meat.

There are recipes for using ground beef or turkey in this book. Ground turkey breast alone, though, will make a meatloaf too dry, so add other kinds of protein to make the dish moister.

Be creative. You can make chopped and ground meat healthier by adding cooked dried beans and dry oatmeal along with an egg or egg whites. Either broil the patties, cook them in a teaspoon of oil in a skillet on top of the stove, or grill them.

Fish are excellent sources of protein. They contain Omega 3, an essential nutrient, especially fatty fish such as salmon. They're relatively low in calories, and they contain the same amount of protein as meat—20 grams per 3 ounces.

There are cautions. Since larger fish feed on smaller fish, the larger fish build up mercury and PCBs in their bodies. These are fish such as canned albacore (white) tuna, shark, swordfish, and king mackerel. Therefore, when you buy and eat fish, choose smaller fish that should have less mercury or the carcinogen PCBs.

Fish that are low in mercury include tilapia, catfish, cod, crab, flounder, haddock, North Atlantic Mackerel, mussels, perch, scallops, sole, canned light tuna, and a few others.

Overall, despite those drawbacks that can be avoided, fish is an outstanding source of nutritious food.

Eggs are good for you. You can boil eggs, bake them as in quiches, or fry and scramble them in just 1 teaspoon oil or an oil spray. The yolks contain multiple micronutrients and one a day doesn't add harmful cholesterol, though 1 egg has about 300 milligrams of cholesterol. Concern about high cholesterol doesn't come from dietary sources like eggs, but from all the saturated and trans fat you eat.

By adding extra egg whites, which have no cholesterol and are high in protein, to a recipe, you're reducing the cholesterol you'd find in a whole egg. And finally, if you prefer, you can use a whole-egg substitute, which is really a combination of egg whites with coloring, spices, salt, onion powder, xanthan gum, and guar gum. Check each brand's ingredients list.

Dried beans are actually a vegetable, and they are a good source of protein as well as many nutrients. You can cook the dried beans yourself (See recipe for cooking dried beans, Chapter 16, "More Healthy, Easy Recipes," page 225.) or buy canned beans, already cooked. (When you use canned beans, be sure you rinse canned beans to remove the excess salt.)

The advantage of cooking dried beans yourself is that you save money and time. Usually you will use only a small portion of the cooked dried beans. What is left over, you can freeze in serving-size or recipe-size containers for future use in making soups, stews, casseroles, salads, extending ground meat, or any number of ways.

Tofu is made from dried soybeans and can be used as a substitute for meat in many recipes. You may not have tried tofu yet, but it is well worth your experimenting with it. (There may be issues in using soybean products for women with breast cancer.)

Nuts and seeds, a good source of protein as well as other nutrients, these are a high-quality snack or an addition to salads and cooked dishes. They make delicious nut and seed butters, are low in saturated fats, and are high in polyunsaturated and monounsaturated fats. Be sure when you buy them that they are salt-free, usually available in the produce section of the grocery store. Roast them yourself for low-cost, high-quality snacks and other uses.

Examples of nuts and seeds you can easily find are: almonds, brazil nuts, cashews, hazelnuts, macadamia nuts, peanuts (really legumes), pecans, pine nuts, pistachios, walnuts, pumpkin seeds, sesame seeds, and sunflower seeds.

Whole Grains

Whole grains play a key role in healthy eating. Most grains can be found at large supermarkets. You can start on the journey of eating whole grains by avoiding white flour in breads, baked goods, and pasta. White flour is a simple carbohydrate and quickly moves into the blood stream, raising our blood levels of sugar and leaving us drained when that level drops, as it will. Instead, buy whole wheat or whole grain products, both of which are complex carbohydrates and enter our bloodstreams more slowly.

Whole grains are intact grains, meaning they are unrefined and the bran and germ haven't been removed. They're a good source of fiber and important nutrients such as selenium, magnesium, and potassium. You will find them in brown rice or popcorn (unsalted and unbuttered!), and in products such as buckwheat pancakes or whole-wheat bread. Whole-grain flours should be stored in an airtight container and placed in the refrigerator. The oils in them will go rancid more quickly than white flour.

When you check the ingredients list of prepared foods, you'll see that most of the so-called whole-grain products contain a portion of white flour. Also, check your Nutrition Facts label on the products. The first ingredient listed should not be white flour but instead be a whole grain, usually those kinds listed below, not white flour.

Whole Grains and Seeds

Amaranth, actually a seed, used as grain or vegetable, originated in the Americas, a flour or cereal.

Barley, one of oldest grains, used whole in soups and other dishes. Look for whole barley.

Brown rice

Buckwheat, not a wheat and not technically a whole grain; look for whole buckwheat.

Bulgur (cracked wheat), quick and easy to cook, used in tabouleh (a cold salad) and as a hot cereal.

Corn, used on or off the cob, as popcorn, and as a ground meal for use in baking. Grits, made from ground corn, is not a whole grain.

Flaxseed, a seed of ancient origins, highly nutritious, found in many foods and cereals.

Millet, used as a flour or cooked whole.

Oats, a flour or flakes used in hot or cold cereal and as an addition to ground meats and some baked goods.

Quinoa, Incan origin, a seed, a complete high protein, gluten free, fast cooking, used like couscous or rice and to make tabouleh. This grain tends to be more expensive than many others.

Rye, a grass grown for its seeds and ground into flour.

Spelt, ancient from many civilizations, a type of flour.

Wheat berries, used as side dish and in salads.

Wild rice, a seed, not a rice, from the Great Lakes in the United States, usually combined with white or brown rice.

Whole wheat flour, white from white wheat, brown from red wheat.

Fats and Cholesterol

Your body needs the good kinds of fats and cholesterol, which are vital to the proper functioning of your cells and brain. You'll find good fats throughout your body, and you won't find them in your arteries, where bad fats do their damage.

Bad Fats

Trans fat is hydrogenated or partially hydrogenated vegetable oil. It is found in solid margarine and in most cookies, cakes, chips, and processed and baked foods. Avoid trans fat. Manufacturers use trans fat because it enables them to store their cookies, cakes, chips, and many other processed foods for longer periods of time..

However, trans fat is even more dangerous than saturated fat that comes from meats and full-fat dairy products because of its ability to easily clog arteries.

Saturated fat is found on and in red meats and whole dairy foods. Although trans fat is a bad fat that clogs our arteries easily and directly, saturated fat is a much larger problem for us because we consume so much of it. You can avoid saturated fat by buying lean meats, such as lean beef, pork, and chicken; by skinning poultry; and by using low-fat or skim milk and all other dairy products.

Good Fats

The average person needs just 4 to 7 teaspoons a day of oil and other fat. Keep that in mind as you choose your oils and fats. Some people use an oil spray to oil pans, limiting the amount of fat in their diets.

Lean meats: To ensure you have good fats, you can use 93% to 96% lean ground beef, lean pork chops with the fat removed, and skinless turkey and chicken breasts.

Low-fat, fat-free, or skim dairy products: Use any low-fat, fat-free, or skim dairy products, including yogurts, sour cream, and reduced-fat cheeses. These are good sources of calcium, protein, and phosphorus, all of which help lower blood pressure.

Vegetable oils: Most vegetable oils are good for you, but not including coconut oil, which can be high in a saturated fats. Good vegetable oils include canola, safflower, sesame, flax, peanut oil, and more. Canola oil has the least amount of saturated and trans fat of any other oil. (Most often, I use canola for cooking and extra-virgin olive oil for salads.)

Omega 3: This is an essential fatty acid, called essential because our bodies need it to function well and because we can't make it without a little help. It is vital in the construction of cell membranes, especially in the eye and brain, as well as in sperm cells and some hormones. Omegas 3s play a role in heart disease protection. If you are getting enough Omega 3 from your diet, you are probably getting enough Omega 6.

Omega 3 is found naturally in fish. Plan on having fish about two times a week in order to get enough. The fish with the highest levels of Omega 3s are fatty fish such as salmon, mackerel, herring, sardines, and tuna. You can use canned or packaged fish, such as dark meat tuna, sardines, or salmon. Solid white tuna may contain high levels of mercury. Check the packages' Nutrition Facts label to be sure there is little or no added salt or bad fat. One of the ways of getting rid or the high salt or bad fat in canned or packaged fish is to rinse it well. Turn the fish out into a colander and rinse, then drain.

Other sources of Omega 3s are walnuts, canola oil and other vegetable oils, ground flaxseed or flaxseed oil, beef, and Brussels sprouts. If you have trouble getting enough Omega 3s from your food, fish oil capsules are a good alternative.

Salt

Processed foods are high in salt and sugar content. They hook you into needing more and more of both of them. Salt, or sodium, increases the likelihood that you will have high blood pressure.

Our bodies need as little as 2400 milligrams, one teaspoon of salt a day, or 1200 milligrams, one-half teaspoon, of salt a day for people over 50 or those at risk for high blood pressure.

The Nutrition Facts labels on packaged foods will list the salt contents by the amount of sodium in each serving. The amount right for you depends on your heart health, body mass, age, and energy expended.

You can cut down on salt by flavoring foods with herbs and spices instead of using the saltshaker. There are a number of salt substitutes, especially those that use a mixture of herbs, such as Mrs. Dash. And you should always buy unsalted foods, adding your own. You will have control, then, and there will be much less salt added.

Sugar

Sugar, or the "–ose" listings, are in the Nutrition Facts label under the category of Total Carbs, then below that Sugars. Your body needs carbohydrates for energy, both in the "fiber" and "sugar" categories. You can easily get both from an apple or another fruit rather than from artificially sweetened foods.

Don't depend on the information you'll find on the Nutrition Facts label regarding sugar because it doesn't let you know whether there's natural sweetness or added sugar. You can better tell the kind of sugar in the product if you check the ingredients list.

But don't try to cut down on sugar by using artificial sweeteners. Some experts believe that artificial sweeteners merely cause you to crave more sweets so you end up eating and drinking more sugars, searching for the satisfaction of eating a sweet.

The officially recommended intake of sugar is 40 total grams per day, not that found naturally in the fruit or vegetables. That adds up to a mere 10 teaspoons of sugar per day.

Though there isn't a direct link between sugar and diabetes, the cause of diabetes can be linked to weight gain with the accompanying fat cells and the increase in inactivity. And much of our weight gain can be linked to far too much sugar along with lack of exercise.

Some nutritionists say we don't need any added sugar in our diets.

Maple syrup, honey, brown sugar—all these are sugars, plain and simple. You're not avoiding the consequences of high sugar in your diet by using these instead of granulated table sugar. You're controlling the amount of sugar in your diet by adding small amounts of each of these.

For example, you can add a tablespoon of maple syrup to your whole-wheat pancakes or a bit of honey to your fruit and yogurt. By adding cinnamon, nutmeg, or vanilla to certain foods, you can cut down on the necessity to sweeten them at all.

High fructose corn syrup is another sugar and might be listed as "corn sugar" or some other innocent-sounding name. Many nutritionists will tell you to avoid high fructose corn syrup, a sugar that is used by manufacturers because it's cheaper than cane or beet sugar. You'll find high fructose corn syrup everywhere these days. High fructose corn syrup might block the messages your body sends that you are full.

Sugars, overall—Don't buy packaged sweetened foods or prepared ice tea. If you need more sweeteners, add your own sugar at the table, that way you can keep track of how much and what you are getting. Adding your own sugar is actually cheaper than buying sweetened packaged foods or ice tea. (If you need to sweeten a cold drink such as tea, keep a solution of sugar water in the refrigerator to add a minimum amount to cold drinks.) Nutritionists recommend learning to drink liquids without any added sugar at all.

Top Ten Power Foods

As reported in the October 2011 issue of *UCLA Division of Geriatrics* newsletter, there are a number of so-called power foods. These are the foods that most experts and dieticians agree that should be eaten more often.

Almonds: Make sure these are unsalted. You can eat these whole as a snack or slivered as a topping for fish, salads, or many other cooked and raw foods.

Apples: One of the most versatile fruits, and you can eat an apple raw out of your hand or sliced in salads, baked in pies or cakes, served as one of many kinds of desserts, sautéed to serve as a side dish, and on and on.

Blueberries: Find these in abundance in the summer months and eat a bowl of them fresh, plain on cereal; baked in a pie, cake or muffins; and used in salads and in countless other ways. Blueberries freeze well. Freeze them when they're abundant and inexpensive. That way you can have them in the winter as well.

Broccoli: This is a versatile vegetable that you can roast, steam, dice, and mix with other foods in stews, egg dishes; or use raw in salads.

Beans: Dried beans, a lean source of protein, can be used in soups, combined with other foods, made into chili or casseroles, or in any number of dishes.

Beets: You can roast, steam, microwave, boil, slice, or add to salads.

Spinach: You can eat this vegetable cooked, mixed with other foods, or raw in salads.

Sweet Potatoes: These are delicious baked, broiled, or boiled, though baked is easiest. Add them cut up to stews and soups.

Wheat Germ: Sprinkle on cereals, hot or cold, and add to meatloaf, stews, or other cooked foods.

Chapter 9

Nutrition Facts Labels

What They Are Really Saying

Read This, Always!
The Nutrition Facts label is your friend. You can learn a lot from reading it, and when you do, you can control the amounts of nutrients and calories you take in every day. Learning to read the label is easy. Check out these Nutrition Facts numbers *before* you buy.

Serving Size: Everything in the product is measured based on what the manufacturer defines as the serving size. It can be deceptive. In other words, if the item says one slice, that means the calories, fat, sodium (salt), and other nutrients are based on that one slice. If you eat two, then you have to double the nutrient count for the two slices you eat to get an accurate count of what you consume.

Calorie count: This is based on the serving size.

Fat, Cholesterol, and Salt: Limit these items: Our bodies need fats and cholesterol to function properly. Just be sure the fats you eat aren't the bad kind. Be careful about adding wrong kinds of fats—trans fats and saturated fats.

Limit your sodium, or salt, to 2400 milligrams per day or to as low as 1200 milligrams per day if you're over the age of 51, black, or have high blood pressure, advises the Mayo Clinic.

Carbs, or Carbohydrates: Carbs have gotten a bad rap among diet gurus because *simple* carbohydrates are found in abundance in baked goods, sweetened goods, sodas, candy, icing, and often in foods that aren't included in a healthy diet. They're linked to weight gain, diabetes, and heart disease. These are the sugar carbs listed on your Nutrition Facts label under Carbohydrates as Sugars.

Complex carbohydrates are essential, not only for energy, but also for brain function.

But your healthy eating plan in this book is loaded with the kind of carbs, *complex* carbs, that increase your energy and include the nutrients you need for leading a healthy life. Complex carbohydrates are essential, not only for energy, but also for brain function. They can keep you alert and vigorous. These are listed on your Nutrition Facts label as Dietary Fiber.

Protein: You don't have to worry that you won't get all the amino acids in proteins because you'll get them if you eat a balanced, varied diet that includes animal sources such as meat, eggs, poultry, fish, milk, milk products; and vegetarian sources such as whole grains, dried beans, rice, and tofu (from soy beans. Most of the world's populations eat vegetable sources of protein).

The question is how much protein, the building block of life, does a body need to repair and maintain itself. Too much protein can lead to kidney damage, high cholesterol if the protein source has one of the bad fats, and other diseases.

You only need two to three servings of protein a day. Here are recommended serving sizes for protein:

- 2 to 3 ounces of cooked lean meat, poultry, or fish (a portion about the size of a deck of playing cards)

- ½ cup of cooked dried beans

- 1 egg, 2 tablespoons of peanut butter, or 1 ounce of cheese

Percent Daily Values: The Daily Values lists the vitamins and minerals that are found in the food.

Sample of Nutrition Facts Label

Nutrition Facts
Serving Size 1 cup (228g)
Servings Per Container about 2

Amount Per Serving

Calories 250   Calories from Fat 110

	% Daily Value*
Total Fat 12g	18%
Saturated Fat 3g	15%
Trans Fat 3g	
Cholesterol 30mg	10%
Sodium 470mg	20%
Total Carbohydrate 31g	10%
Dietary Fiber 0g	0%
Sugars 5g	
Proteins 5g	
Vitamin A	4%
Vitamin C	2%
Calcium	20%
Iron	4%

* Percent Daily Values are based on a 2,000 calorie diet. Your Daily Values may be higher or lower depending on your calorie needs:

	Calories:	2,000	2,500
Total Fat	Less than	65g	80g
Saturated Fat	Less than	20g	25g
Cholesterol	Less than	300mg	300mg
Sodium	Less than	2,400mg	2,400mg
Total Carbohydrate		300g	375g
Dietary Fiber		25g	30g

For educational purposes only. This label does not meet the labeling requirements described in 21 CFR 101.9.

Chapter 10

Munching!

Snacks for a Healthy Diet

Snack Away!

Your secret weapon for a healthy life is to be ready with healthy foods.

Healthy food in your cabinets and refrigerator won't do you any good if you still are looking for a ready-to-eat snack that is high in fats, sugars, and salt. Snacks can make or break your healthy eating plan.

> *[Dark chocolate] makes you smile.... That's a very small bite of dark chocolate, though.*

Snacks are so important to your health that they are a regular part of the healthy eating plan menus. Snacks keep you from getting famished and binging to satisfy the cravings that sneak up on you, and healthy snacks can add to your daily nutrition needs.

Stock your pantry and refrigerator with some easy, ready-to-eat foods such as those listed below. Snack regularly so you can ward off a binge attack.

Cut-Up Veggies and Fruit with Sources of Protein

You can have all sorts of healthy veggies and even fruit sitting in your fridge, but neither you nor your family will grab it for a snack if it's not ready to go. Instead, you will grab a bag of chips or some other ready-to-eat snack, most likely loaded with sugar, salt, and fat.

Make it easy for everyone to be healthy by washing and cutting the fruit and veggies into bite-size pieces. Keep those pieces in plastic containers or resealable zip-lock bags so they're always ready to eat. Have pieces of reduced-fat cheese, 8-ounce containers of yogurt, small containers of cottage cheese, and peeled hard-boiled eggs ready in the refrigerator. Store ready-to-eat nuts and dried fruit in the cabinet.

Fruit and veggies with a source of protein, such as those listed in Chapter 8, "Healthy Eating Nutrition," pages 45-55, are extremely satisfying and give you energy to last until the next meal without the feeling that you're famished.

Trail Mix

Make your own trail mix from nuts; dried fruit; and low-fat, low-sugar cereal. Put your mix in a plastic container, and when you're ready to snack, you can just grab and go. Or you can munch on small amounts while watching TV, reading, or just hanging out.

One type of trail mix combines nuts, dried fruit, and cereal. You can make your own by combining equal parts roasted, unsalted nuts, your favorite kind; and dried fruit, such as raisins. You could also add some sugar-free, fat-free dry cereal such as Kellogg's All-Bran, Bran Buds, Kashi Go-Lean, Barbara's Shredded Spoonfuls, Nabisco's Mini Shredded Wheat without the sugar coating, Post's Grape Nuts, and others of your choosing.

Mix the ingredients and store in plastic lidded containers in your pantry. Chopped roasted walnuts and raisins, for example, make a quick and healthy snack.

Granola or Energy Bars

Some granola bars are really candy bars. Look for granola or energy bars that are high in protein, somewhat low in sugars and fats, barely sweet, and crunchy. They can be an alternative to cookies and cake. Buy granola or energy bars made of whole grains, dried fruit, and nuts.

Cooked Chicken Breast

This is a surprise! Cut up some leftover chicken breast, put it in a plastic container, and you have a great protein-rich snack. You can also add a little lite mayonnaise and some raisins to the cut-up chicken. Good for energy when you feel low.

There are other ways to eat this treat: Wrap some of the mixture in a lettuce leaf or in a tortilla with whatever cut-up fresh veggies you have on hand, if you wish. When you add a little cheese to the tortilla along with some vegetables, you have made a quesadilla.

As always, be creative with your food. It's fun that way, delicious, and healthy.

Other Snack Ideas

- Frozen grapes, frozen bananas

- Orange segments, broccoli or cauliflower florets, grape tomatoes, and other fruits and vegetables of your choice—with a protein

- Hard-boiled eggs

- Salad leftovers, including tuna, chicken, fish, dried beans, or cheese

- Hummus as a dip with whole wheat crackers or pita wedges and with celery and other cut-up firm vegetables

- Low-fat or fat-free plain yogurt, flavored yogurt, or Greek yogurt, along with cut-up banana, strawberries, or other fruit

- Smoothies that include fruit, yogurt, milk or "milk" of your choice, and juice

- Sunflower seeds, salt-free, with fruit

- Tuna with cut-up apples

- Cooked shrimp with vegetables

- Sargento string cheese light with a vegetable or fruit

- Polaner all-fruit preserves with crackers and reduced-fat cheese (Smuckers also has some all-fruit, but be careful that the total sugar does not sabotage your healthy eating plan.)

- Rice cakes, low-salt, spread with sources of protein such as peanut or other nut butters

- Corn chips, baked, no- or low-salt, with protein dip such as hummus (recipe, page 192)

- Peanut or other nut butters with whole grain or graham crackers

- Pickles or olives. Be careful of too much salt or sugar in these items. Have a protein source such as chicken salad with this snack.

- Dark chocolate, 60% to 80%, satisfies and a little goes a long way. Just a serving, about the size of a quarter, can reduce blood pressure by about 30 percent. Dark chocolate is high in antioxidants and can help reduce the incidence of arteriosclerosis and blood clotting, and contribute overall to a reduction in heart attacks and cholesterol levels. It makes you smile, too. That's a very small bite of dark chocolate, though.

Chapter 11

Tools

Make Cooking Easy

Keep your kitchen and the tools you use to prepare your food as simple as possible. Many labor-saving devices frequently aren't actually labor saving. For example, the food processor. It is a lot of extra work to put it together and then clean it. I prefer the old-fashioned way of chopping with a knife and cutting board. But if you like these labor saving devices, then please use them.

There are several tools that are easy to use and that I recommend. You do not have to buy expensive tools. A less expensive model gets the job done very well.

Blender: This can do a great deal of the work a food processor can do, except make piecrust and bread. It is certainly a good tool for making smoothies and shakes, pureeing foods, and mixing soups.

Immersion or handheld blender: This is a wonderful tool, and you can use it instead of the stand-up blender. You take the hand-held device to the food instead of taking the food to the device. It is especially good for blending and pureeing soups in the saucepan and pureeing fruit for yogurt. Some immersion or handheld blenders allow you to grate cheese and chop garlic.

Food processor: This is a very popular device, but it is not actually necessary. They are expensive and an effort to set up and clean for tasks that can be done simply in a blender or on a cutting board.

Slow cooker or Crockpot: These devices are good for stews and many other dishes. A slow cooker or Crockpot can help you by having your food ready when you walk in the door after work, though you'll have to start the dish before you leave. Follow the manufacturer's directions for cooking.

Toaster oven: This appliance can save you electricity and will make cooking tasks easy and quick. And it doesn't heat up the kitchen during the summer.

Microwave: This appliance saves time and your personal energy as well as that from the electric company. Microwaves are useful for reheating foods and steaming vegetables.

Instant read thermometer: This instrument is not totally necessary but a convenience.

Timer: These can be found on stoves and microwaves, but a separate, stand-alone timer is useful.

Pots or Saucepans: You'll need several sizes that range from small to large, some with covers, and they will be used for cooking rice, grains, pasta, soups, stews, and vegetables.

Steamer: Today these are small, aluminum devices that unfold to fit in the bottom of a saucepan, just above the low water line. Put water in the saucepan so it's below the steamer, place the food in the steamer, cover the saucepan, boil the water, and steam.

Skillet: The best for cooking many items is the non-stick skillet, both large and small, with and without a cover. It will be used for sautéed food, eggs, and many other dishes.

Skillet, cast iron: You will use a cast iron skillet often. For baking cornbread and making smaller dishes, you'll use an 8-inch cast iron skillet. For cooking pancakes and larger items, you'll need a 12-inch cast iron skillet.

Cookie sheet: Many of your foods will be baked on a rimmed cookie sheet, usually lined with aluminum foil for easy cleanup.

Baking pans and dishes, including loaf pans: Whenever you bake foods—such as vegetables, breads, and fruits—you'll use these in various sizes.

Mixing bowls: These come in many sizes. You'll use them all.

Measuring cups and spoons: You'll need a variety for making many dishes. You'll need the kinds that measure liquid as well as those used for dry ingredients.

Spatulas: Non-metal spatulas are used for lifting out cooked items from non-stick pans and metal are used for working with iron or metal skillets. Metal spatulas are also useful for loosening baked goods from their pans.

Scrapers: These tools are usually rubber and convenient for removing all the ingredients from mixing bowls.

Spoons: You will use large size cooking spoons for stirring and dipping foods out of saucepans.

Spoon, slotted: This is a really handy implement for draining and removing cooked items from saucepans. Usually a large size is best.

Spoons, wooden: These are convenient to have for stirring food while it is cooking and are useful for breaking up ground meat while it's cooking.

Whisk: You can use a whisk to beat liquids and eggs. Whisks incorporate air into the liquid.

Tongs: These help you pick up foods like spaghetti, pasta, green beans, broccoli, and other difficult-to-grab foods.

Grater: Usually a box grater is most useful, though a straight-sided one can be just as useful, especially for small grating tasks.

Kitchen shears: These are basically scissors and are useful for cutting meats, herbs, and vegetables instead of using a knife. They make chopping and cutting quick and easy. And you can use them for opening packages.

Knives: These are important items and you'll need and use them in various sizes and styles. You'll need them serrated for cutting breads, large and sharp ones for slicing meats and cutting vegetables and fruit into small sizes, small and sharp ones for smaller jobs. You'll use knives frequently, so choose the ones you feel comfortable with. Do not buy an expensive, sharp knife unless you are adept with your hands and can avoid cutting off a finger.

Cutting board: This is essential and makes cutting and slicing tasks much easier. A non-wood cutting board cleans easier.

Colander: You'll use this for a lot more than draining cooked spaghetti. It's good for rinsing fruit, draining and rinsing canned beans, and so much more.

Strainer: This item is useful for straining liquids to get the lumps or solid pieces out or for sprinkling flour over the bottom of a pan.

Plastic containers: Various sizes from small to large. Useful for storing refrigerated, frozen, or dry foods as well as for taking lunches and snacks to work, school, and on outings.

If You Need a Little Extra Help

Electric can opener: This handy device opens cans quickly without any effort needed for turning the handle.

Rubber cloths: These work to loosen tight caps. By draping a cloth or other rubber item such as a rubber glove over the lid, you gain leverage and can open the formerly tight lid.

Jar opener: By applying this device over the lid of a jar and giving it a little twist, you can easily screw off the lid without the force you'd usually apply to such a task.

Reacher: With one of these nearby, you can reach items that were formerly out of your reach. Carefully grab the item with the reacher and pull it toward you. Do not try to lift heavy items from a height. They work best when you need to drag something toward you from below or from a height not much higher than you.

Kitchen tools and utensils with large rubber handles: By adding easy-to-hold larger rubber handles, many kitchen utensils have become much less difficult to hold and operate. These are excellent tools for the compromised or handicapped person. Look for them where utensils are sold.

Chapter 12

The Healthy
Eating Plan

Explained

Research into the subjects of healthy eating, obesity, and the associated diseases led me to understand that healthy eating doesn't end with food choices, but must include exercise and stress relief. Thus, a busy person can use this entire book with its information on exercise and stress relief, but most especially the recipes that were made for them—cooking with ease and simplicity. And this is absolutely not a gourmet cookbook!

Like most of us, you probably want to be healthy but don't know where to begin. You think it's too much trouble. But the goal of this book is to make living and eating extremely simple. So even you can become healthy!

You'll discover that cooking at home is both cheaper and a great deal healthier than going out or picking up some fast food. You will find there's added benefit to eating at home—cooking it the way you like it, having your friends and family with you, and knowing you're helping yourself become healthier.

How to Begin

You might not be able to use this healthy eating plan all at once. Some people like to follow menus and recipes as they are given; some don't. Some days you may find it harder to follow the plan than others.

You can pick and choose the recipes you like. Look in the Recipe Index for recipes and foods you'd like to have. Some of the recipes are marked as Super Easy. Go to those when you need some extra help or don't have the time or energy to cook.

You can pick and choose the ingredients in each recipe, depending on what's on sale, your individual preferences, and your time available. There's no perfect way to cook! You'll see you have a choice with many ingredients.

If you choose the ingredients that suit you, it's very important that you choose what's healthy. By now you know the rules.

Exercise and relaxation are such important parts of this healthy lifestyle plan. Please don't leave them out as they are not demanding and they are vital parts of the three levels of health. The whole point of this book is to create a healthful living plan that is so simple it can become a natural part of your everyday life.

Quick Review of the Principles

Follow the principles behind this plan. That means every meal will have fruits and vegetables, whole grains, and lean protein. It means every meal omits "bad" fats, too much salt and sugar, and white flour based foods.

Reality Eating

Let's face it. Many of us won't have time to make the breakfasts in these menus. Nor have the time to pack a healthy lunch. There are two steps you can take to ensure you remain on a healthy diet despite lack of time and energy.

First, make sure your quick meals, for either breakfast, lunch, or dinner, follow the basic rule, which is to always have healthy, low-fat protein; always have fruits or vegetables, more than you'd usually have; and always have a whole grain.

That's relatively easy if you pay attention to it, even when you go out to eat. But don't go to a fast food outlet and expect you'll get a healthy meal, even if they have oatmeal, for example. Their oatmeal is packed with sugar, fat, and a lot of calories.

Second, and this may sound much more difficult than it really is, get up fifteen minutes early! That's all the time you need to get together a healthy breakfast and pack a healthy lunch. Just fifteen minutes.

SPEEDY MEAL IDEAS: WHEN YOU'RE ON THE RUN

For Breakfast

- Take a slice of reduced-fat cheese. Wrap a slice or piece of whole grain bread around it. Add fruit—a whole apple, a bunch of grapes, or a banana. Bring your coffee, tea, or "milk" in a non-spill container. You're ready to go!

- Take a peeled, hard-boiled egg. Add unsalted whole grain crackers. Add fruit and coffee, tea, or a "milk" to the package.

- Spread natural peanut butter or other nut butter, on whole grain bread. Fold. Add fruit and coffee, tea, or "milk."

- Put about ½ cup roasted, unsalted nuts in a baggie. Take whole grain crackers, fruit, and coffee, tea, or a "milk."

For Lunch or Light Meal

- Place a handful of washed lettuce pieces in a container, add cut vegetables, fruit, and some nuts that you have on hand. Put ¼ cup salad dressing in a small lidded jar to add to your salad later. Or you can put your salad dressing on the bottom of the container and toss to mix when you're ready to eat.

- Place peeled, hard-boiled egg and grape tomatoes in a small container. Pack whole grain crackers or bread in a baggie. Take milk or water.

- Place leftover cooked and sliced chicken breast in a container. Add lettuce leaf pieces. Place ¼ cup salad dressing in a small lidded jar. Pack whole grain bread or crackers in a baggie. Add milk or water.

For Snacks

- Put cut-up vegetables and fruit into serving-sized bags, ready to grab when you need them.

- Keep low-fat, low-salt cheese sticks in the refrigerator.

- Keep packages of non-refrigerated fruit cups, low-sugar and high-protein energy bars, instant plain oatmeal, cereal, low-salt pretzels, and other healthy snacks in your pantry for quick pick-me-ups.

For Dinner or the Main Meal

- You can heat up leftovers.

- You can use leftovers in quick soups or salads.

- You can make sandwiches from meats, eggs, cheeses, even tofu.

- You can make a stir-fry by adding a leftover wholegrain to a heated, oiled skillet and adding pieces of your leftovers: meats, beans, nuts, vegetables, and an egg to bind it all together. Stir with a spatula until heated through. Serve,.

FOR DESSERT

- Serve ½ cup fresh, frozen, or canned fruit with ½ cup frozen yogurt, ice milk, or fat-free yogurt. Place ½ plain graham cracker on side.

HINTS FOR BUSY COOKS AND THOSE WHO NEED EXTRA HELP

- When you get home from a long day out or when you're so tired you don't think you can lift a pan to cook anything, try a quick snack such as a carton of yogurt, a small container of Almond Milk, a glass of milk with some honey stirred in, or some other quick pick-me-up that doesn't sabotage your healthy eating plan. You'll gain a second wind and will be able to feed yourself well.

- The Super Easy recipes are labeled in the text so you can find them quickly. Look for them when you're tired, don't want to think about cooking, or need some extra help.

- Be sure your pantry and refrigerator are stocked with foods from the Basic Shopping List, Chapter 6, "Stock Your Kitchen with Delicious, Healthy Food," pages 28-39. That will save you a lot of time, energy, and money.

- You can always buy frozen or canned vegetables and fruits, especially when they're on sale. But you must make sure they don't contain added salt, sugar, or fat. They are handy to have on hand for those days when you don't want to go to the grocery store or farmers market and for when you need them NOW.

- You'll still get your day's worth of nutritious vegetables and fruit by using frozen or canned. You know they're nutritious because they're packed immediately after harvesting from the fields.

- You can double or triple a recipe, so you won't have to remake the whole recipe the next time you use it for another meal. I love leftovers. They mean I cook less often and know I'm eating healthy food. All you have to do is refrigerate or freeze and thaw, and reheat a serving-size portion in the microwave, oven, or toaster oven.

- Use a trick busy chefs use and it works just as well for the rest of us. It's called *mise en place*, French for "putting in place" or "everything in place." Before you begin, take out your supplies that you will need for the recipe, and then get your ingredients out so they're ready to use. Put them close by the place where you're going to mix, cut, stir, and cook. You'll find it's all much simpler this way.

Chapter 13

Menus! Recipes!

The Healthy Eating Plan!!

The goal in these recipes is to help you lose weight gradually and permanently and for you to remain healthy. You'll find it's easy to keep the food healthy. You'll keep the kitchen and cook cool in the spring and summer, and in fall and winter you'll warm your soul as well as your body. Compared to going out to eat, these homemade foods are a lot cheaper and better for you and your family. And believe me, they're actually easy to make. There's not a gourmet recipe in this book, but you'll be creating, not just buying and consuming.

The ingredients can be changed or eliminated. If you can't eat tomatoes or dairy, for example, leave those ingredients out. The recipe won't be significantly changed and you'll be able to eat it.

Spring and Summer

Bountiful!

The "Healthy Eating Plan" for spring and summer includes menus and recipes for six days that are geared for warmer months. With these recipes, you won't cook as much as you would in the cooler fall and winter months.

In both seasons, the resulting recipes are simple and healthy. The spring and summer recipes feature many of the season's fruits and vegetables. You can add and substitute any that you find available for sale or in a nearby garden.

Early spring vegetables include asparagus, new potatoes, and new lettuce. Most treasured among the mid-summer vegetables are vine-ripened tomatoes and summer squash, both yellow and zucchini. And you'll find okra and corn later in the season.

The earliest of the fresh fruits are strawberries, though you can find them in US markets most times of the year. Then come the blueberries, and you can follow the season of blueberry ripening when the first harvest comes from Florida and then ends up somewhere in the upper Midwest. Along with the blueberries come blackberries and raspberries. South American and Central American berries are also available later in the year.

The stone fruits, such as peaches, apricots, and plums, are in recipes for bowls of fresh fruit, cobblers, crisps, and baked dishes. In this book, the recipes are low-sugar, low-fat, and all without crusts.

Spring and Summer

Day 1 Menus

BREAKFAST

➤ Whole Grain Cold Cereal[1] with Milk, Low-Fat or Skim, or "Milk"[2] of Your Choice, and Fresh Fruit

➤ Coffee or Tea[3], with Sweetener[4] and/or Fat-Free Half-and-Half Cream[5]

[1]Choose your favorite whole grain cereal such as Wheaties, Cheerios, All Bran, Kashi Go Lean, and many more. Read the Nutrition Facts label to make sure there is no added sugar or fats. You can add fruit, nuts, ground flax seed, and other healthy foods.

[2]Any kind of "milk" is fine with this meal plan. That includes instant, soy, goat, rice, almond, cow, sheep, hemp, oat, coconut, flax seed, and others. Keep in mind that non-dairy milk often has less protein and calcium than dairy milk and may have added sugar and be high in fat (coconut milk).

[3]Caffeine found in coffee or tea, not herb tea, has some benefits as well as drawbacks. It is suspected of reducing the tendency to acquire Type 2 diabetes, Parkinson's disease, and dementia, as well as lessen the likelihood of experiencing certain cancers, heart rhythm problems, and strokes. There are drawbacks to drinking too much caffeine—sleeplessness, raised blood pressure, heart burn, and frequency of urination.

[4]Do not use artificial sweeteners. Some nutritionists think they cause you to crave more sweets. Instead, use minimal amounts of sugar or honey.

[5]Some people like half-and-half cream with their coffee or tea. You can find a fat-free half-and-half that is quite good with those drinks or even with cereals and fruit. Fat-free half-and-half doesn't have much nutritional value, so keep its use to a minimum.

MAIN MEAL

➢ Salmon with Brown Sugar, Balsamic Vinegar, and Light Soy Sauce Marinade

➢ Brown Rice or Couscous

➢ Baby Lettuce[1] Salad with Scallions and Seasonal Vegetables with Bottled or Homemade Salad Dressing

➢ Baguette, Whole Wheat[2]

➢ Blueberries or Strawberries with "Milk"

[1]Choose your favorite lettuce. The darker the lettuce leaves are, the more nutrients they have.

[2]The term "whole wheat" as used in these recipes is interchangeable with any number of whole grain products. According to the Food and Drug Administration, by using the whole grain, you have access to "intact, ground, cracked … kernel, which includes the bran, the germ, and the inner-most part of the kernel (the endosperm)." This means that the endosperm, the part of the seed that contains multiple nutrients, is intact. Look for barley, buckwheat, bulgur, corn, millet, rice, rye, oats, sorghum, wheat, and brown rice.

LIGHT MEAL

➢ Garden Bean Salad with Fresh Vegetables

➢ Whole Wheat Pita

SNACKS

You may choose a snack from the list in Chapter 10, "Munching!," pages 59-62. Make a snack of your own using the guidelines on snacks or leftovers. Snacks are important. Don't let yourself get too hungry and thus overeat. A snack with some protein as well as the good kind of carbohydrate gives you energy when you begin to sag.

➢ Nuts and Raisin Mix

➢ Hummus with Vegetables

Day 1 Recipes

BREAKFAST

Whole Grain Cold Cereal with Milk, Low-Fat or Skim, or "Milk" of Your Choice, and Fresh Fruit

Serves 2

INGREDIENTS

> 1-2 cups whole grain cold cereal, your choice (See the Nutrition Facts label for serving size. Note the number of calories in the manufacturer's "serving size" that is often not related to the way we eat. Also make sure there's little added sugar or fats.)
>
> 1-2 cups low-fat or skim milk, or "milk" of your choice
>
> 1 cup fresh fruit, depending on what's in season
>
> 2 teaspoons sugar or honey, if necessary

METHOD

Place one serving, or about ½ to 1 cup, of cereal into each of two bowls. Pour in ½ to 1 cup milk or "milk" of your choice. Add ½ cup fruit, cut up if necessary, and ½ teaspoon sugar.

Coffee or Tea

Serve coffee or tea, if using, and add low-fat or skim milk, "milk" of your choice, or fat-free half-and-half cream and sugar or honey to taste, keeping the sweetener to a minimum.

MAIN MEAL

Salmon with Brown Sugar, Balsamic Vinegar, and Light Soy Sauce Marinade
Serves 2

INGREDIENTS

1 pound salmon fillet, fresh caught or farm grown (This amount leaves leftovers.)

1 tablespoon brown sugar

1 tablespoon Balsamic vinegar or other vinegar

1 tablespoon light soy sauce

METHOD

1. Raise oven shelf to about 6 inches below the broiler coils. Pre-heat oven to broil. Cover rimmed cookie sheet with aluminum foil. Place salmon fillet, skin-side down, on the cookie sheet.

2. In a small bowl combine the brown sugar, vinegar, and light soy sauce. Stir until the sugar is dissolved. Pour part of this mixture by the tablespoonful over the salmon. Let sit for about 15 minutes. Reserve the remaining mixture to add to the cooking salmon and to serve over rice or couscous.

3. Place cookie sheet with salmon under the broiler and cook on the first side for about 4 to 6 minutes. Remove the cookie sheet from the oven, turn the salmon over with a spatula, and spoon more marinade over the fish. Insert cookie sheet back into the oven and broil another 3 to 4 minutes, or more. The flesh should be firm, flaky, and opaque.

4. Remove cookie sheet from the oven and scrape off or remove the skin from the fillet.

5. There are four servings in a 1-pound fillet. Serve the leftover marinade in a small bowl for the rice or couscous. Serve half the cooked salmon fillet for dinner for two. Reserve the other half of the salmon fillet for another meal.

Brown Rice

Brown rice is available frozen or in easy-to-make boxes. When you use the prepared rice, you'll find that the preparation effort is about the same as using the recipe below, but the rice won't be as nutritious and probably more expensive. Follow the directions on the package for the desired number of servings.

This, however, is an easy recipe and much cheaper than prepared rice. If you make more than you need for a meal, you can freeze or refrigerate the remainders for future meals, saving you a step. All you have to do is heat in the microwave.

Serves 4-6

INGREDIENTS

1 cup long-grain brown rice

1 ½ cups water or vegetarian, chicken, or beef broth, canned or boxed, or mixture of the two

METHOD

1. Add brown rice to medium size saucepan with water, broth, or mixture of the two.

2. Bring to a full and vigorous boil. Immediately turn down the heat to a simmer and cover saucepan. Check two or three times in the first minute to make sure the liquid is not boiling over.

3. Set timer to 45-50 minutes and lift lid only when the time is up. Check whether the rice has absorbed all the water and that the rice is fluffy.

4. If that is the case, remove the saucepan from the heat and leave the lid on until ready to serve. If the rice is not yet ready and there is still liquid to be absorbed by the rice, leave the covered saucepan on low heat for another 5 minutes, repeating till done.

5. Leftover rice can be frozen for future use. Place serving-size amounts of the cooked rice in resealable plastic bags or covered plastic containers. Freeze. To defrost, place the frozen rice in a loosely covered bowl, using a paper towel or wax paper, in a microwave and heat on high for about 1 to 1 ½ minutes.

Couscous

Couscous is small pasta from North Africa. You can buy instant whole wheat couscous. It goes well with many main dishes and is very easy to make. It makes a good salad by adding chopped or shredded vegetables. For making couscous, follow the package directions or those below.

Serves 2

INGREDIENTS

1 teaspoon extra virgin olive oil or canola oil

½ cup instant, packaged whole wheat couscous

¾ cups boiling water; vegetarian, chicken, or beef broth with reduced salt and fat; or a mix of the two

1 teaspoon dried parsley or ½ cup fresh chopped parsley, optional

METHOD

1. Bring water and/or broth to a boil in a medium saucepan. Add couscous.

2. Immediately cover and remove from heat. Allow the couscous to sit undisturbed for 5 to 10 minutes.

3. Fluff gently with a fork. Serve.

4. To use for other dishes, refrigerate or freeze leftover couscous in serving-size resealable plastic bags or containers. Reheat by placing the couscous in a bowl, loosely covered with a paper towel or wax paper, and heat in the microwave for 1 to 1½ minutes.

Baby Lettuce Salad with Scallions, Seasonal Vegetables, and fruit with Bottled or Homemade Salad Dressing

Serves 2

INGREDIENTS

2 cups baby lettuce leaves, packaged and pre-washed, or washed lettuce of your choice

2 stalks scallions, sliced into ½ inch pieces, including the green parts. Remove roots and dead ends. You may also use any other kind of chopped onion.

1-2 cups washed seasonal vegetables such as chopped summer squash or zucchini, chopped or sliced tomatoes, sliced mushrooms, packaged shredded carrots, or other vegetables of your choice

¼ cup washed and chopped fruit such as grapes, apples, strawberries, blueberries, or the fruit of your choice

1 tablespoon bottled low-sodium (salt), low-fat salad dressing such as Italian or Caesar or Homemade Salad Dressing (recipe below)

Salt and pepper to taste

METHOD

1. Tear lettuce into pieces or use pre-washed packaged lettuce pieces. Place torn lettuce, onions, and sliced or chopped vegetables and fruit in a big bowl.

2. This salad is improved by adding vegetables and fruits, but you can reduce or eliminate any or all of them. Add dressing.

3. Toss to cover the lettuce, vegetables, and fruit thoroughly with the dressing. Serve on small plates or beside salmon.

Homemade Salad Dressing

Salad dressing, either bottled or homemade, is used not only for salads but also as a marinade for meats and other dishes. It's kept in the refrigerator for future use.

Serves 4-6, or more

INGREDIENTS

     1 cup extra virgin olive oil or canola oil

     1-2 tablespoons vinegar (Balsamic, apple cider, white, your choice of vinegar, or lemon juice) or bottled pure lemon juice. Adjust ratio of oil to acid ingredients according to your preference.

     2 tablespoons water

     1 teaspoon Dijon mustard (optional, helps emulsify the dressing as well as add a tangy taste.)

     1 teaspoon sugar or honey

     Salt and pepper to taste

METHOD

1. Mix all salad dressing ingredients in a jar or other container. Shake to mix.

2. You can keep bottled pure lemon juice on hand for the times you don't have fresh lemons.

The ultimately simple salad dressing that I use in a pinch

1. For 2 servings pour 2 teaspoons vinegar (Balsamic, apple cider, white, or you choice of vinegar) on salad ingredients in a bowl, keeping the vinegar or lemon juice to a minimum. You can always add more if you wish, but it's hard to take away the vinegar.

2. Then pour about ½ cup canola oil or extra virgin olive oil over salad. Toss. Sprinkle salt to taste over the salad. Taste and adjust ingredients as needed. Serve.

Baguette, Whole Wheat

Buy one entire loaf of whole wheat baguette. On a cutting board, slice diagonally across the length into 2- to 3-inch pieces. Set aside 2 slices for one meal for 2 servings and freeze the remainder in a resealable plastic bag for future meals. Reheat on warm, not toast, in a toaster oven.

Blueberries or Strawberries with "Milk"

Serves 2

INGREDIENTS

1 pint carton fresh blueberries or strawberries, or 1 box or bag frozen blueberries or strawberries (other berries can be used in this recipe)

½-1 cup low-fat or skim milk, fat-free half-and-half cream, or "milk" of your choice

1 teaspoon honey, if desired

METHOD

1. Wash blueberries or strawberries or partially defrost frozen blueberries or strawberries. If using fresh strawberries, remove stem end and cut into bite-size pieces. Place ½ cup berries into each of two small bowls, reserving the remainder for cereal, salads, or other use.

2. Pour ¼ to ½ cup low-fat or skim milk, fat-free half-and-half, or "milk" of your choice over berries and add honey if necessary. Serve.

LIGHT MEAL

Garden Bean Salad with Fresh Vegetables
Serves 4-6

INGREDIENTS

1 15-ounce can of beans such as navy, white, cannelli, or pinto. You can use 1½ cups cooked dried beans, from 16-ounce package, recipe page 225

Choose among the following: (This salad is best the more vegetables you use.)

½ cup carrots, shredded

½ cup celery, chopped

½ cup bell pepper, chopped

½ cup onion, chopped,

½ cup other vegetables on hand,

1 tablespoon low-fat, low-sodium bottled Italian or Caesar salad dressing or 1 tablespoon Homemade Salad Dressing, recipe page 83

3-4 washed lettuce leaves, your choice, or 2 cups packaged pre-washed lettuce

METHOD

1. Pour canned beans into a colander. Rinse well. Drain. Rinse and drain again. Add the rinsed and drained beans to a large bowl. *Or* use 2 cups cooked dried beans, drained, from 16-ounce package.

2. Add your choice of prepared vegetables, fresh or packaged.

3. Place in the refrigerator for about 30 to 45 minutes to cool. When you remove from the refrigerator, add salad dressing. Mix well. (If using commercial bottled salad dressing, test for acidity. Add oil to cut the tartness.) Serve over lettuce leaves that have been spread on plates.

Whole Wheat Pita

Place a whole pita in a toaster oven on warm for 5 to 7 minutes. Remove and cut into 6 to 8 wedges. Serve beside Garden Bean Salad.

SNACKS

Nuts and Raisin Mix

Serves 2 for several days

INGREDIENTS

1 cup roasted nuts from a bag or container of raw unsalted nuts such as peanuts, almonds, walnut pieces, almonds, or other favorite nuts

1 cup dried raisins

METHOD

1. Buy raw, unsalted nuts in the produce section of your grocery or online from a nut vendor. Roast nuts by spreading them on a rimmed cookie sheet and baking in a 350-degree oven for 8 to 9 minutes, being sure they don't overcook or burn. Remove from oven and allow to cool. Store any unused nuts in a plastic container, resealable bag, or glass jar for future use.

2. Mix 1 cup raisins and 1 cup roasted nuts in a bowl. Place in a covered container.

3. Snack on ½ cup mix at a time. Reseal container in between snacks.

Hummus with Vegetables

You can buy prepared hummus or make your own hummus by following the recipe, page 192.

Serves 2 for several days

INGREDIENTS

1 container prepared hummus. There are several flavors, such as red pepper and garlic. Make sure it is low salt.

1 cup or more firm vegetables from pre-washed packages such as bell pepper, broccoli, carrots, celery, and other firm vegetables, sliced or chopped into dipping-size pieces, about 2 inches. You can also prepare your own.

METHOD

Dip cut vegetables into hummus and eat a total of ½ to 1 cup vegetables with dip at a time. Cover leftover hummus and place vegetables in plastic bags or containers and keep refrigerated for future use.

Day 2 Menus

Breakfast

➤ Smoothie with Fresh Fruit and Yogurt

➤ English Muffin, Whole Wheat or Whole Grain

➤ Coffee or Tea

Main Meal

➤ Honey-Soy-Sauce-Vinegar Marinated Baked Chicken

➤ Steamed Shredded Vegetables

➤ Couscous, Whole Wheat

➤ Baguette, Whole Wheat

➤ Strawberries or Other Seasonal Fruit with Vanilla Yogurt and Graham Cracker

Light Meal

➤ Leftover Salmon Fillet Sandwiches on Whole Wheat Bread

➤ Salad with Lettuce, Fruit, Nuts, and Vegetables

Snacks

➤ Cottage Cheese with Fruit

➤ Peanuts

Day 2 Recipes

BREAKFAST

Smoothie with Fresh Fruit and Yogurt
Serves 2

INGREDIENTS

About 1 cup frozen fruit, such as banana, pitted peach, blueberries, hulled strawberries, and so forth. You may freeze fresh fruit for this recipe or buy frozen at the grocery store. You may also use fresh, washed fruit.

Approximately ½ cup low-fat or skim milk, or "milk" of your choice

1 cup plain yogurt or Greek yogurt, low-fat or fat-free

1 teaspoon honey or to taste, if necessary

1 English muffin, whole wheat or whole grain

1 teaspoon soft-tub margarine[1]

> [1]Soft-tub margarine should contain no trans fat or saturated fats that you often find in processed foods, red meat, and butter. When you can, use oils instead. Fats in themselves are not bad for you. It's the kind of fats that matters.

METHOD

1. Before freezing, cut or break larger frozen fruits, such as banana, into 1- to 2-inch pieces. After they are frozen, place the frozen fruit, milk, yogurt, and honey in a blender. You may use a handheld blender with the ingredients in a bowl large enough so that the smoothie does not spill over the edge.

2. Add milk as needed to make smoothie pourable. Push down the ingredients while blending with a rubber spatula. Adjust amount of honey to taste, blending at each addition, but keep honey at a minimum. Pour in tall glasses and drink or eat with a spoon.

3. Toast English muffin halves or other whole grain bread and serve with soft-tub margarine that contains no trans fat or saturated fats or with olive oil that has been solidified by cooling in the refrigerator.

4. Serve coffee or tea, if desired. Add fat-free half-and-half cream and sweetener, if necessary.

MAIN MEAL

Honey-Soy-Sauce-Vinegar Marinated Baked Chicken

"My husband was extremely impressed about how moist the chicken was with a gorgeous coloring on the outside!! And it was just too easy." Nicole Hayward

This is delicious. Easy to make and worth repeating again and again. I first learned how to make this on a camping trip. That's how easy it is.

Serves 4

INGREDIENTS

    1 skinless chicken breast or 3-4 skinless thighs or combination

    1 tablespoon extra virgin olive oil or canola oil

    1 tablespoon honey

    2 teaspoons reduced-salt or lite soy sauce

    2 teaspoons vinegar, Balsamic, apple cider, white, or your choice

METHOD

1. Trim fat off chicken pieces and remove skin. Place in a zip-locked baggie.

2. In a small bowl, mix together the honey, soy sauce, and vinegar. Stir until the honey is dissolved. Add the mixture to the bag, zip closed, and move the chicken pieces around with your

hand so the mixture covers them all. Place in the refrigerator for 30 minutes to an hour.

3. After the chicken has marinated, preheat the oven to 400 degrees. Line a rimmed cookie sheet or roasting pan with aluminum foil.

4. Place the pieces on the cookie sheet or in the pan and put into the preheated oven. Roast for about 25 minutes, adding marinade to the chicken periodically.

5. When the chicken is done, not exuding pink juice when pressed, remove from the oven and serve with couscous and a salad.

Recipe tested by Nicole Hayward

Couscous, Whole Wheat

Reheat 2 servings of couscous, previously prepared from recipe on page 81, by placing frozen couscous into a small bowl, covering loosely with a paper towel or wax paper, and heating in a microwave on high for 1 to 1 ½ minutes. Remove and carefully open, as it may be steamy, and test for warmth. Place in a serving bowl or on plates.

Steamed Shredded Vegetable

You can find a variety of shredded vegetables in the produce department. You can steam or microwave them. These vegetables add significantly to your daily needs for vegetables, which are about 5 or 6 ½ servings a day, or more, according to the Harvard School of Public Health. One package of these shredded vegetables will last for a while.

Serves 2

INGREDIENTS

1 or more packages shredded vegetables, such as carrot, cabbage, and broccoli

1 tablespoon water

½ teaspoon salt

METHOD

1. Remove a total of 1 cup shredded vegetables from the packages and place in a microwave-safe bowl. Add about 1 tablespoon water. Cover loosely with a paper towel or wax paper. Microwave for 1 minute for crispy vegetables and for 1 ½ to 2 minutes for softer vegetables. Check texture periodically.

2. You can also steam these vegetables by placing them in a small saucepan fitted with a steamer basket. Add water up to the bottom of the steamer and bring to a boil. Cover and steam for 3 to 5 minutes. Check periodically for doneness.

3. Sprinkle with minimum salt and pepper to taste and serve.

Baguette, Whole Wheat

Use frozen pre-cut baguette pieces. Warm in a toaster oven for about 2 to 3 minutes or until thawed and warm. Do not toast. Serve with extra virgin olive oil or soft-tub margarine. (You can "harden" olive oil by placing some in an open-mouth jar and refrigerating until "hardened.")

Strawberries or Other Seasonal Fruit with Vanilla Yogurt and Graham Cracker

Serves 2

INGREDIENTS

1 8- or 16-ounce carton fresh strawberries, 1 bag or box frozen strawberries, unsweetened, or 1 can sliced fruit and packed in fruit juice. Other fruit may be substituted.

1 teaspoon sugar, or to taste, optional

1 8-ounce carton vanilla yogurt, low-fat or fat-free

½ whole graham cracker, low-fat, no trans fat

METHOD

1. Rinse strawberries or other fruit thoroughly if using fresh. Drain. Hull strawberries by cutting off green stem ends and slice into bite-size pieces. Put about ½ cup sliced strawberries into small bowls, with minimum sugar, and 1 tablespoon vanilla yogurt. Place ¼ whole graham cracker beside the strawberries.

2. If using frozen strawberries or other fruit, partially defrost, cut into bite-size pieces, and serve as above.

3. If using canned, remove the fruit from the fruit juice and place about ½ cup into small bowls. Discard the juice. Serve as above.

4. Reserve remaining fruit for cereals or snacks and the vanilla yogurt for fruits or snacks.

LIGHT MEAL

Leftover Salmon Fillet Sandwiches on Whole Wheat Bread
Serves 2

INGREDIENTS

½ pound leftover broiled, marinated salmon (from recipe on page 79)

2 slices whole wheat or whole grain bread

2 teaspoons lite mayonnaise

METHOD

1. Toast bread, if desired, or warm. Spread with lite mayonnaise on each cut side.

2. Place salmon fillet on one piece of the bread and top with the second. Cut sandwich into half. Serve.

Salad with Lettuce, Fruit, Nuts, and Vegetables
Serves 2

INGREDIENTS

2 cups lettuce, from a head of your preferred lettuce
or from a container of pre-washed lettuce leaves

1 cup vegetables, cut up, sliced, or shredded. Choose
from carrots, bell peppers, onions, tomatoes,
squashes, and many more that are available
in the spring and summer. Use pre-washed
packaged vegetables or prepare your own.

1 tablespoon roasted nuts, no salt, optional

½ cup fruit, such as blueberries, strawberries, grapes,
or fruit of your choice, optional

2 teaspoons or more salad dressing, either bottled,
such as low-fat, low-salt Italian or Caesar or
from the Homemade Salad Dressing, recipe
page 83

METHOD

1. Place torn lettuce leaves, vegetables, nuts, and fruit cut into
   bite-size pieces in a medium-size bowl. Add salad dressing.
   Toss and serve on small plates or beside sandwich.

SNACKS

Cottage Cheese with Fruit

Use ½ cup low-fat or fat-free cottage cheese with cut-up fruit such as strawberries, blueberries, peaches, fruits on hand, other fresh in-season fruits, or canned or frozen fruits.

Peanuts

Buy a container of dry-roasted, salt-free peanuts. Serve ¼ to ½ cup at a time as a snack.

Day 3 Menus

BREAKFAST

➤ Poached Eggs on Whole Grain Bread

➤ Fruit

➤ Milk, Low-fat or Skim, or "Milk" of Your Choice, or Water

➤ Coffee or Tea

MAIN MEAL

➤ Greek-Style Chickpea Salad on Lettuce

➤ Baguette, Whole Wheat, or Crackers

SUPER EASY

LIGHT MEAL

➤ Leftover Honey-Soy-Sauce-Vinegar Marinated Baked Chicken Salad with Fruit

➤ Whole Grain Crackers

SUPER EASY

SNACKS

➤ Plain Yogurt with Fruit

➤ Whole Wheat Crackers with Peanut Butter and Low-Fat or Skim Milk, or "Milk" of Your Choice

Day 3 Recipes

BREAKFAST

The following items in this breakfast are placed in order of preparation. Try to finish the eggs last so they will be hot when you serve them.

Serves 2

Fruit

Choose fruit that is available to you, whether hulled strawberries, blueberries, sliced pitted peaches, or any number of spring and summer fruits, fresh, canned, or frozen, with no added sugar. Place about ½ cup fruit into a small bowl and serve at the same time you're serving the eggs and bread.

Whole Grain Bread

You can use a bread of your choice. English muffins go well with poached eggs. Toast the bread before you begin to poach the eggs so you will have it ready to lay the cooked eggs on top. Spread each piece with 1 teaspoon soft-tub margarine or olive oil that has been hardened by refrigerating.

Poached Eggs

Serves 2

INGREDIENTS

2 eggs, large

Water, to cover the eggs

1-2 teaspoons vinegar, optional

METHOD

1. Heat about 1 to 2 cups water in a medium-sized nonstick skillet until water is hot but not boiling. Add vinegar, if using. Vinegar helps the whites to coagulate.

2. Gently break eggs, one at a time, into a small bowl, and then slide each one into the hot water so they are not touching. If necessary, use a smaller skillet and cook eggs one at a time.

3. Spoon hot water over the eggs so the top turns white as it cooks and the yellow firms but is not hard, or cook to taste.

4. With a slotted spatula, lift the eggs, one at a time onto the toasted bread on which you have spread soft-tub margarine or hardened olive oil.

5. Serve milk, low-fat or skim, or "milk" of your choice, or water with breakfast. Also serve coffee or tea, if using, adding very little sugar or honey, fat-free half-and-half cream, or a "milk" of your choice.

Main Meal

Greek-Style Chickpea Salad on Lettuce
"This recipe was very good." Linda Prospero
Serves 2-4

INGREDIENTS

- 1 15-ounce can chickpeas (or beans of your choice)
- 1 teaspoon powdered or dried minced onion, ⅓ cup scallions or onion of your choice, chopped
- 2 teaspoons powdered or dried minced garlic or 1 clove garlic, peeled and chopped
- ½ cup cucumber, peeled, seeded, and chopped, or sliced into thin disks, optional
- ½ cup shredded vegetables such as carrots, bell peppers, and broccoli, as available in produce section of grocery store
- 2 teaspoons dried mint or 3 tablespoons fresh mint leaves, chopped
- 3 tablespoons feta cheese, crumbled, or dry curd cottage cheese, low-fat or fat-free
- 3 tablespoons chopped pitted black olives, available in small cans, or Kalamata olives, chopped, if available
- 2 teaspoons dried parsley leaves or 2 tablespoons fresh parsley leaves, chopped
- 1-2 tablespoons bottled salad dressing such as low-salt and low-fat Italian or Caesar or Homemade Salad Dressing, recipe page 83
- Salt and pepper to taste, kept to a minimum
- 2-4 lettuce leaves, your choice, washed and patted dry with paper towels

METHOD

1. Place canned chickpeas or other canned cooked dried beans in a colander. Rinse well and drain. Repeat.

2. In a large bowl, place rinsed chickpeas, onion, cucumber, if using, vegetables of your choice, mint, feta or cottage cheese, and parsley. Toss well.

3. Pour either bottled or homemade dressing onto chickpeas and vegetables, toss to cover well, chill, and serve over washed lettuce leaves arranged on plates with choice of warmed baguette or crackers.

Leftover salad can be kept in a closed container in the refrigerator for 3-4 days for future use. This is good for a light meal or snack.

Recipe tested by Linda Prospero

LIGHT MEAL

Leftover Honey-Soy-Sauce-Vinegar Marinated Baked Chicken Salad With Fruit
Serves 2

INGREDIENTS

Use ½ pound or approximately 1 cup of cooked chicken from previous day

1 cup fruit such as grapes or cut-up apple

METHOD

Serve cold as a fruit salad, with fruit such as grapes or cut-up apples. Add whole grain crackers of your choice.

SNACKS

Plain Yogurt with Fruit
Serves 2

INGREDIENTS

1 cup plain yogurt or plain Greek yogurt, low-fat or fat-free

½ cup fruit such as hulled and sliced strawberries, blueberries, sliced bananas, or fruit of your choice, fresh, canned, or frozen, with no added sugar

1 teaspoon honey, as needed

METHOD

Place ½ cup yogurt in small bowls. Top with ¼ cup prepared fruit and honey. Serve.

Whole Grain Crackers with Peanut Butter and Low-Fat or Skim Milk, or "Milk" of Your Choice

Serves 2

INGREDIENTS

2 whole grain crackers or 1 large cracker, halved

1 tablespoon peanut butter, natural, with no added fats or sugar

1 8-ounce glass low-fat or skim milk, or "milk" of your choice

METHOD

Spread crackers with peanut butter. Serve with milk or "milk" on the side.

Day 4 Menus

BREAKFAST

➤ Whole Grain Bagel with Low-Fat Cream Cheese or Neufchatel and Fruit Jam or Honey

➤ Fruit, Your Choice

➤ Milk, Low-Fat or Skim, or "Milk" of Your Choice

➤ Coffee, Tea, or Other Acceptable Beverage

MAIN MEAL

➤ Summer Pizza with Mozzarella Cheese, Bell Peppers, Tomatoes, and Spinach Leaves

➤ Blueberries or Other Fruit of Your Choice, with Vanilla Ice Milk or Frozen Yogurt

LIGHT MEAL

➤ Leftover Greek-Style Chickpea Salad with Whole Wheat Pita

SNACKS

➤ Hummus and Vegetable Pieces (crudités)

➤ Soybeans (Edamame)

Day 4 Recipes

BREAKFAST

Whole Grain Bagel with Low-Fat Cream Cheese or Neufchatel and Fruit Jam or Honey

Serves 2

INGREDIENTS

2 small or one large whole wheat bagel

(You can use another type of bread such as rye, pumpernickel, English muffin, or crackers such as Rycrisp, Kashi, or Wasa. Be sure you check the label to see if the product is actually whole grain.)

2 teaspoons honey or low-sugar fruit jam (Often this kind of fruit jam is made with concentrated apple juice, which can be high in sugars. Check the amount of sugars per serving on the label.)

1 tablespoon low-fat cream cheese or Neufchatel cheese

METHOD

1. If possible, take cream cheese out of refrigerator about 10 to 20 minutes before using to bring to room temperature.

2. Divide or slice bagels and warm or toast as desired. Spread each half with ½ tablespoon cream cheese or Neufchatel and 1 teaspoon honey or jam, as desired.

Fruit

Place ½ cup chosen and prepared fruit in each of 2 small bowls. Add ½ teaspoon sugar or honey, as desired. Serve.

Beverages

Pour milk, or "milk" of your choice, or water into glasses. Serve coffee or tea, if desired. Add minimum amount of sugar, honey, your choice of milk or fat-free half-and-half cream to coffee or tea. Serve beside bagel or other whole grain bread or cracker and fruit.

MAIN MEAL

Summer Pizza with Mozzarella Cheese, Bell Peppers, Tomatoes, and Spinach Leaves

"Good!" Steven Risi

Serves 2-4

INGREDIENTS

- 1-2 whole wheat pitas for ½ pita per person
- 1-2 tablespoons or more from jar pizza sauce, such as Prego
- 1 ½ cups shredded, reduced-fat mozzarella cheese
- 1-2 tomatoes, sliced, or 5-7 grape or cherry tomatoes, halved
- 1 cup fresh baby spinach leaves, chopped or torn, from pre-washed packaged baby spinach leaves
- ½ cup onion, chopped or slivered
- ½ cup bell pepper, from pre-washed packaged, or from whole bell pepper, seeded, pith removed, and cut into strips
- 2 tablespoons fresh oregano, if available, or 2 teaspoons dried oregano leaves
- 1 clove garlic, peeled and chopped, or ½ teaspoon garlic powder or minced dried garlic

**Salt and pepper, to taste, using a minimum amount
    of salt**

2 tablespoons grated Parmesan cheese

METHOD

1. Preheat oven to 450 degrees or toaster oven to bake. Place pitas on an aluminum-foil-lined cookie sheet or toaster oven tray and bake for about 5 minutes until just beginning to brown. This step will give the pitas some structure to hold the vegetables and cheese without becoming saturated with moisture.

2. Remove from the oven and spread pizza sauce on top of each pita, followed by the shredded mozzarella cheese.

3. Cover the cheese with the tomatoes, spinach, onion, bell pepper, oregano, and garlic, spreading items evenly over the surface. End by sprinkling the Parmesan cheese over all.

4. Return to oven and bake for another 10-20 minutes or until the pita edges are light brown and the cheese is fully melted. Cut each pita pizza in half and serve.

Recipe tested by Steven Risi

Blueberries or Other Fruit of Your Choice, with Vanilla Ice Milk or Frozen Yogurt

Serves 2

INGREDIENTS

1 cup fresh blue berries or frozen blueberries or other berries or fruit of your choice

1 cup vanilla ice milk or frozen yogurt

METHOD

1. Wash fresh blueberries or partially defrost frozen blueberries. Prepare other fruit, if using. Place ½ cup blueberries or other fruit into each of two small bowls. Top each with ½ cup vanilla ice milk or frozen yogurt. Reserve remaining fruit for future use.

LIGHT MEAL

Leftover Greek-Style Chickpea Salad with Whole Wheat Pita

Serves 2

INGREDIENTS

2 cups leftover Greek-Style Chickpea Salad

1 whole wheat pita

METHOD

1. Measure the remaining Greek-Style Chickpea Salad, recipe on page 100. If you do not have 2 cups, add torn lettuce and feta cheese or dry cottage cheese (low-fat or fat-free and low-salt) to make the 2 cups.

2. Heat a whole pita in a toaster oven on warm, not toast, or a 350-degree oven for 5 to 7 minutes. Remove, divide in half, and with your fingers pull the pita open.

3. Into each half, insert salad. If the pita won't open, use as a wrap, with about ½ to 1 cup salad. Serve on each of two plates.

SNACKS

Hummus and Vegetable Pieces (Crudités)
Serves 2

INGREDIENTS

Assortment of firm pre-washed packaged vegetables or cut vegetables from what you have on hand

1 container of prepared hummus, low-salt, or homemade hummus, recipe page 192

METHOD

1. Use pre-washed, packaged vegetables, or firm vegetables, such as broccoli, celery, and carrots cut into strips for dipping into the hummus. Serve about ½ to 1 cup vegetables each person.

2. Dip each piece of cut vegetable into the hummus.

Soybeans (Edamame)

Serve ½ cup shelled soybeans (fresh or frozen) per person. They can be eaten as is or with a minimum of salt added.

Day 5 Menus

SUPER EASY

BREAKFAST

➤ Toasted Cottage Cheese on English Muffin with Low-Sugar Fruit Preserves or Jam

➤ Fruit, Your Choice

➤ Low-Fat or Skim Milk, or "Milk" of Your Choice

➤ Coffee, Tea, and Water

MAIN MEAL

➤ Omelet with Onion, Bell Pepper, Tomatoes, and Mushrooms with Herbs and Parmesan Cheese

➤ Baguette, Whole Wheat

➤ Spiced Peach Goodie

LIGHT MEAL

➤ Pasta Salad with White and Black Beans, Spinach, Tomato, Herbs, and Feta Cheese and Salad Dressing

➤ Whole Grain Crackers or Bread

SUPER EASY

SNACKS

➤ Favorite Cereal with Low-Fat or Skim Milk or "Milk" of Your Choice

➤ Reduced-Fat Cheese with Whole Grain Crackers

Day 5 Recipes
BREAKFAST

Toasted Cottage Cheese on English Muffin with Low-Sugar Fruit Preserves or Jam
Serves 2

INGREDIENTS

2 tablespoons low-fat or fat-free dry-curd cottage cheese

1 English muffin, whole grain, halved

2 dashes cinnamon, ground, optional

2 teaspoons low-sugar fruit preserves or jam of your choice

METHOD

1. Spread 1 tablespoon cottage cheese on each half of an English muffin and dust lightly with powdered cinnamon, if desired.

2. Place under broiler in oven or toaster oven and broil until the edges of the bread begin to turn brown.

3. Remove with a spatula and place on each of two plates. Serve with low-sugar fruit preserves or jam on the side.

Fruit

Select favorite in-season fresh, frozen, or canned fruit. Be sure frozen or canned fruit is sugar-free. Wash and slice if needed. Place ½ cup into each of two small bowls. Add bit of sugar or honey if needed.

Low-Fat or Skim Milk, "Milk" of Your Choice, or Water and Coffee or Tea

Serve milk or water with coffee or tea, adding sugar, milk or fat-free half-and-half cream only as necessary to the coffee or tea.

MAIN MEAL

Omelet with Onion, Bell Pepper, Tomatoes, and Mushrooms with Herbs and Parmesan Cheese

"This is an easy weekend breakfast or brunch dish using veggies on hand." Ruth Porter

Serves 2

INGREDIENTS

2 teaspoons extra virgin olive oil or canola oil

1 teaspoon powdered or dried minced onion or ½ cup onion, chopped

½ cup pre-washed packaged bell pepper or bell pepper, seeded, pith removed, and chopped

½ cup grape or cherry tomatoes, halved, or ½ cup from 14.5-ounce can diced tomato, drained (save liquid for making soup)

1 4-ounce can sliced mushrooms or ½ cup sliced mushrooms, white or your choice

1 teaspoon dried herbs, such as parsley, basil, or oregano or ¼ to ½ cup fresh herbs, chopped

3 eggs or egg substitute to equal 3 eggs

2 teaspoons water

2 tablespoons grated Parmesan cheese

Salt and pepper, to taste, using a minimum of salt

METHOD

1. Place oil in a large non-stick skillet on medium heat. Add vegetables and fresh herbs, if using. Sauté until limp while preparing eggs. Remove from heat if cooking too quickly.

2. Break whole eggs into a small bowl or pour egg substitute into a small bowl. Beat eggs with a fork until mixed. Add water and mix again. If using dried herbs, add to the mixture and stir.

3. Pour egg mixture into heated skillet with sautéed vegetables. Stir gently as the eggs cook, mixing all ingredients.

4. Cook until eggs reach desired doneness, and then remove immediately from heat and sprinkle Parmesan cheese over top. Add salt and pepper to taste.

5. Serve on two plates with toasted or warmed whole wheat baguette or whole grain bread.

Recipe tested by Ruth Porter

Spiced Peach Goodie

"The recipe was very easy, and it was great over ice cream. Nutmeg adds to the overall flavor of the dish." Matt Lardie

Actually this is a peach pie without the crust, and the "Goodie" method can be used with other fruits such as blueberries, blackberries, plums, and other stone fruits.

Serves 2-4

INGREDIENTS

> ½ teaspoon canola oil
>
> 3-4 peaches, ripe; 1 container or 1 pound frozen; or 1-2 cans, unsweetened and drained; or enough peaches to make 2-3 cups (Fresh peaches make the best Peach Goodie.)
>
> Juice of ½ lemon or 1 tablespoon bottled pure lemon juice
>
> ½ cup light brown sugar, loosely packed
>
> ¼ teaspoon dried ground nutmeg, optional
>
> ½ teaspoon ground cinnamon
>
> 2 tablespoons cornstarch

METHOD

1. Preheat oven to 350 degrees. Prepare a pie plate or an 8 x 8 baking pan by oiling with canola oil

2. Prepare peaches or other fruit. If using fresh peaches, halve, remove pit, and cut into approximately ½ inch slices. Peel if desired.

3. If using frozen, allow to defrost before using in the recipe. If using canned, measure about 2 cups for this recipe, reserving liquid for future use.

4. Place peaches or other fruit in a large bowl.

5. Squeeze juice from fresh lemon, if using. Remove seeds. Sprinkle fresh or bottled lemon juice over peaches.

6. In a small bowl, add brown sugar, nutmeg if using, cinnamon, and cornstarch. Mix well and then stir the dry ingredients into fruit.

7. Place peaches mixed with all ingredients in the oiled pie plate or baking pan and put into preheated oven.

8. Bake for about 30 to 40 minutes or until peaches are bubbly. Remove and allow to cool slightly before serving with about ½ cup vanilla frozen yogurt, ice milk, or yogurt. This dish can also be served cold.

9. Save remaining Spiced Peach Goodie in the refrigerator for snacks or future desserts.

Recipe tested by Matthew Lardie

LIGHT MEAL

Pasta Salad with White and Black Beans, Spinach, Tomato, Herbs, and Feta Cheese, and Salad Dressing

"*This is a beautiful salad when placed in a large glass bowl.*" *Elaine Bauman*

Serves 2-4

INGREDIENTS

1 cup of cooked whole wheat pasta, such as farfel (bow ties), spiral, or rotini, or the pasta style you prefer. (You can boil a 8- or 16-ounce package of whole wheat pasta and reserve the leftover for future use in serving-size containers or plastic bags.)

1 15-ounce can white beans, such as navy, drained and rinsed

1 15-ounce can black beans, drained and rinsed, or
   canned beans of your choice or 2 cups cooked
   and drained dried beans from a 16-ounce
   package, recipe page 225

1 teaspoon powdered or dried minced onion or ¼
   cup chopped onion

1 cup fresh spinach leaves, washed, or pre-washed
   packaged spinach, torn into bite-size pieces

1 tomato, quartered, or 5 halved grape or cherry
   tomatoes

2 teaspoons dried herbs, such as basil or sage, your
   choice, or ½ cup chopped fresh herbs

1 cup crumbled feta cheese or shredded Parmesan
   or mozzarella cheese or shredded or crumbled
   cheese of your choice

2 tablespoons salad dressing, such as bottled low-fat
   and low-sodium Caesar or Italian or Homemade
   Salad Dressing, recipe page 83

Salt and pepper to taste, starting with a minimum
   amount of salt

METHOD

1. If cooking a 16-ounce package of dry pasta, bring about 4 to 6 quarts of water to a boil. Quickly add spirals, rotini, or chosen pasta and return to boil. Cook for about 10-12 minutes, according to package directions, or until *al dente,* barely soft but not too soft. Drain.

2. Or follow directions for cooking small amounts of dry pasta in a frying pan, page 225.

3. Place about 2 cups cooked pasta in the refrigerator to cool. (Package remaining cooked pasta for future use in serving-sized, resealable plastic bags or containers.) In about half an hour, remove the cooling pasta from the refrigerator and place in a large bowl.

4. Add ½ cup each rinsed and drained white and black beans, or 1 cup beans of your choice. (Reserve leftover beans for snacks or future use.) Add onions, spinach, tomatoes, and herbs. Toss. Add salad dressing, and toss well.

5. Serve with whole grain crackers or warmed bread with extra virgin olive oil or canola oil on the side.

Recipe tested by Elaine Bauman

SNACKS

Favorite Cereal with Low-Fat or Skim Milk or "Milk" of Your Choice

A good and easy choice for a snack is a small bowl of your favorite whole grain cereal with the low-fat or skim milk or a "milk" of your choice and some fruit on top. As always, be sure the cereal is whole grain and contains no added sugar or fats.

Reduced-Fat Cheese with Whole Grain Crackers

Serve a slice of any reduced-fat cheese on top of a whole grain cracker.

Day 6 Menus

BREAKFAST

➢ Cheese, Fruit, and Nuts with Toasted Whole Grain Bread
➢ Low-Fat or Skim Milk or "Milk" of Your Choice, or Water
➢ Coffee, Tea, or Water

MAIN MEAL

➢ Fish Fillets with Tomato, Onion, Capers, and Black Olives
➢ Brown Rice, Couscous, or Other Whole Grain or Pasta
➢ Lettuce, Tomatoes, Nuts, and Fruit
➢ Baguette, Whole Wheat
➢ Angel Food Cake Slices with Chocolate Frozen Yogurt

LIGHT MEAL

➢ Pasta with Tomatoes and Parmesan Cheese
➢ Simple Salad
➢ Whole Wheat Baguette or Crackers

SNACKS

➢ Whole Grain Crackers with Peanut Butter and Banana
➢ Leftover Garden Bean Salad

Day 6 Recipes
BREAKFAST

Cheese, Fruit, and Nuts and Toasted Whole Grain Bread
Serves 2

INGREDIENTS

½ cup cubed or sliced reduced-fat cheese, such as reduced-fat Swiss or part-skim mozzarella

½ cup roasted, salt-free nuts, such as walnuts, almonds, or others of your choice

1 cup prepared fruit, such as washed blueberries, hulled strawberries, pitted stone fruits, or frozen or canned fruit with no added sugar

METHOD

1. Place ¼ cup cubed cheese or 1 slice cheese with ¼ cup roasted nuts on each of two plates. Put ½ cup prepared fruit into each of two small bowls.

2. Serve with low-fat, skim milk, or "milk" of your choice, or fat-free half-and-half cream and/or water. Place your choice of coffee, tea, or water on the table.

MAIN MEAL

Fish Fillets with Tomato, Onion, Capers, and Black Olives

"I love the flavor the capers added. The dish was really easy and tasty. I like the fact that it cooks all in one skillet and is done in about 30 minutes." Carol Wills

Serves 4-8

INGREDIENTS

1 tablespoon extra virgin olive oil or canola oil

1 teaspoon powdered or minced dried onion or ½ cup onion, chopped

1 teaspoon garlic powder or minced dried onion or 1 clove garlic, peeled and chopped

1 14.5-ounce can tomatoes, diced, any flavor

1 tablespoon capers, optional

2 tablespoons canned black olives, sliced and drained, optional

Pinch crushed red pepper flakes, optional

1 teaspoon dried parsley or 2 tablespoons fresh parsley, chopped

1 pound raw fish fillets such as tilapia, snapper, sea bass, grouper, sole, or flounder. Tilapia is inexpensive. You can also look for flash-frozen fish, especially tilapia.

Juice of ½ lemon, 1 tablespoon bottled pure lemon juice, or 1 teaspoon vinegar

METHOD

1. Heat oil in large nonstick skillet over medium heat. Add fresh onion and sauté until tender, if using fresh.

2. Add fresh garlic, if using, and sauté for 1 minute more. Stir in canned tomatoes with juice.

3. At this point, add powdered garlic and onion, if using, and parsley. Add red pepper flakes, capers, and black olives, if using.

4. Cover and simmer on low for about 10 minutes. (This dish tastes best if you use most of the listed ingredients.)

5. Remove cover and add tilapia fillets. Drizzle the lemon juice or vinegar over the fillets and spoon the sauce over them.

6. Re-cover and simmer for another 10 to 15 minutes, depending on the thickness of the fillet. The fish is done when it flakes easily with a fork.

7. Serve over about ½ to ¾ cup cooked brown rice, couscous, or other pasta.

Recipe tested by Carol Wills

Brown Rice, Couscous, or Other Whole Grain or Pasta

See recipes for brown rice and couscous, page 80-81. If you have leftovers to reheat, place 2 servings of brown rice, couscous, or other pasta on a loosely covered plate or bowl and heat in the microwave for 1 to 1½ minutes.

Lettuce, Tomatoes, Nuts, and Fruit
Serves 2

INGREDIENTS

2 cups pre-washed packaged lettuce leaves, or 2-3 leaves from head of lettuce, your choice

5 grape or cherry tomatoes, halved

1 tablespoon walnuts, almonds, or nuts of your choice, chopped or slivered

1 tablespoon grapes, halved, or fruit of your choice

2 teaspoons bottled salad dressing such as Caesar or Italian, with little or no added salt, fat, or sugar, or Homemade Salad Dressing, recipe page 83

Salt and pepper to taste

METHOD

1. Place lettuce, torn into bite-sized pieces, into a bowl. Add halved tomatoes, chopped or slivered nuts, and halved grapes or fruit of your choice.

2. Add salad dressing. Toss to cover all ingredients with salad dressing. Add salt and pepper. Taste and adjust seasonings.

3. Serve on small plates. Reserve remainder of this salad to serve with Light Meal.

Whole Wheat Baguette

If you have baguette slices in the freezer, remove 2 and reheat on warm in a toaster oven for about 4 to 5 minutes, or until warmed and defrosted. Serve with extra virgin olive oil, if desired.

If you do not have any remaining cut pieces, slice a whole wheat baguette across the length into 2- to 3-inch pieces. Serve 2 pieces with Main Meal and place extra pieces in resealable plastic bags and freeze for future use.

Angel Food Cake Slices with Chocolate Frozen Yogurt

It's hard to get easier than this, and it's healthy, too. The problem is that you'll have the whole angel food cake to tempt you. You can save yourself by cutting the remainders into serving-size pieces, placing them in a freezer-safe zip-lock bag, and hiding them in the freezer along with the chocolate frozen yogurt container.

Serves 2

INGREDIENTS

2 small slices each about 2 inches thick from a whole angel food cake

122

1 cup chocolate frozen yogurt from a container of frozen yogurt

METHOD

1. Place 1 slice of the angel food cake on each of 2 plates. Top with ½ cup frozen chocolate yogurt. Serve.

2. You can choose other flavors of the frozen yogurt or substitute flavored low-fat or fat-free yogurt.

SUPER EASY

LIGHT MEAL

Pasta with Tomatoes and Parmesan Cheese

"Very tasty!!! A quick favorite to enjoy every time." Carol Cantrell

Serves 2-4

INGREDIENTS

1 16-ounce package whole wheat pasta such as rotini, spiral, or your choice (You will use only 2 cups of the cooked pasta and freeze the remainder in serving-size containers for future dishes. Also see the method for cooking small amounts of pasta in a skillet, page 226.)

1-2 fresh tomatoes, chopped, or about 1 cup grape or cherry tomatoes, halved (Ripe, juicy tomatoes preferred.)

½ cup grated or shredded Parmesan cheese. Add more as needed.

1 teaspoon dried basil or 4-5 fresh basil leaves, chopped

Salt and pepper to taste, salt kept to a minimum

2 slices warmed whole wheat baguette or crackers

METHOD

1. About an hour before you wish to serve, bring about 4-6 quarts water in a large pot or saucepan to a boil. Quickly add spirals, rotini, or chosen whole wheat pasta and return to a boil, uncovered. Cook for about 10-12 minutes, according to package directions, or until *al dente,* barely soft but not too soft.

   (You can test the pasta for doneness while it is cooking and almost done. With a long fork pull some pasta from the water, cool slightly, and test by eating it. If it crunches, it's not done. Let it cook for another minute or two, then test again.)

2. Drain cooked pasta in a colander set in the sink.

3. Place about 2 cups cooked pasta in the refrigerator to cool. (Save the remainder in a serving-sized containers and place in the freezer for future use. Reheat by placing on a plate or in a bowl, covering loosely, and microwaving for about 1 minute.)

4. After about 30 to 40 minutes, remove the cooling pasta from the refrigerator, and place in a large bowl. Chop or dice the fresh basil or measure 1 teaspoon dried basil. Add chopped or halved tomatoes, Parmesan cheese, and basil to the cooked pasta in a serving bowl. Add salt and pepper, keeping salt to a minimum.

5. Toss, taste, and adjust seasoning. Serve with leftover salad and about 2 slices warmed whole wheat baguette or crackers.

Recipe tested by Carol Cantrell

SNACKS

Whole Grain Crackers with Peanut Butter and Banana

Serves 2

INGREDIENTS

1 or 2 whole grain crackers with no trans fats, such as Rycrisp, Kashi, Wasa, or the like

1 tablespoon natural peanut butter, with no added sugar or fats (other than the naturally occurring peanut oil), on the 2 pieces of cracker

METHOD

1. Divide the selected cracker so there are 2 pieces or use 2 small crackers.

2. Cover with banana slices.

3. Serve with milk, low-fat, skim, or "milk" of your choice, if desired.

Leftover Garden Bean Salad

Serve ½ cup of Leftover Garden Bean Salad into each of two bowls.

Fall and Winter

Cool Months

Warm and Cozy

As the days get cooler, we love to turn to the kitchen, or at least to the foods that comfort us. In this section, you'll find recipes that use the oven and that warm the soul—all easy to make and savor. The stews and oven-baked foods are, like the spring and summer dishes, always very easy to make.

You'll find winter vegetables—acorn squash and its numerous relatives, turnip greens and other greens, radishes, cauliflower, mushrooms, onions, and more. This is a good time for chili and stews. Fruits include the citrus, figs, grapes, apples, and pears. As always, you can easily use canned or frozen vegetables and fruit. It all depends on your time and budget. And desserts for fall and winter don't have to be unhealthy to be good.

All these cool weather recipes are healthy, even though they are almost sinfully delicious. And, I promise you, none are gourmet!

Day 1 Menus

BREAKFAST

➤ Oatmeal[1] with Raisins and Walnut Pieces[2]

➤ Milk, Low-Fat or Skim, of "Milk" of Your Choice

➤ Unsweetened Applesauce or Navel Orange Segments

➤ Coffee or Tea

> [1]There are other hot cereals that are delicious, such as Wheatena, Roman Meal hot cereals, Irish oatmeal, oat bran, and other whole grain hot cereals. You can make it easier for yourself by cooking for 3-4 days at a time and saving servings for the following days in plastic containers. reheat loosely covered in a microwave for about 1 to 2 minutes to serve. Make sure the hot cereals are whole grain and contain no added sugar or fats. To cook, follow the package directions.

> [2]Any number of nuts and seeds can be used here as well as walnut pieces. They are low in saturated fats and high in polyunsaturated and monounsaturated fats. Some good choices for hot cereals are walnut pieces, sliced almonds, pecans, and seeds such as flax and sunflower kernels. See Chapter 8 on "Healthy Eating Nutrition," the section on "Nuts and Seeds," page 49.

MAIN MEAL

➤ Turnip or Mustard Greens[1]

➤ Black-Eyed Peas

➤ Brown Rice

➤ Cornbread

➤ Baked Pears

> [1]Mustard greens can be substituted for turnip greens. You may use packaged pre-washed, chopped greens or frozen greens. If you use freshly harvested greens from the garden, the preparation is important. They must be carefully washed under running water until there is no longer any grit, which is the soil. Cut the large rib from the leaves and tear into small pieces.

LIGHT MEAL

➤ Easy Basic Soup

➤ Cornbread

SNACKS

You may choose a snack from the list in Chapter 10, "Munching! Snacks for a Healthy Diet," pages 59-62, make a snack of your own using leftovers or the guidelines on snacks, or use the suggestions below. Snacks are important so that you don't let yourself get too hungry and thus overeat. A snack with some protein as well as the good kind of carbohydrate gives you energy when you begin to sag.

➤ Banana, Peanut Butter,[1] and Whole Grain[2] Bread or Crackers

➤ Apple and Cheese

[1]Peanut butter or other nut butters naturally have oil that rises to the top of a newly opened jar. You can drain this oil from the jar before serving or mix it into the nut butter. Some of the right kinds of fats are both necessary and good for you and the working of your body.

[2]According to the Food and Drug administration, by using the whole grain you have access to "the intact and unrefined, ground, cracked or flaked fruit of the grains." This means that the endosperm, which is a part of the seed and is packed with nutrients for the developing plant, is intact. Look for barley, buckwheat, bulgur, corn, millet, rice, rye, oats, sorghum, and wheat whole grains.

Day 1 Recipes
BREAKFAST

Oatmeal with Raisins and Walnut Pieces
2 Servings

INGREDIENTS

> **1 cup old-fashioned, quick, or *plain* instant oatmeal (If using instant, choose the kind that has no added sugar or fats and follow package directions before adding raisins and walnut pieces.)**
>
> **1-1½ cups water (more water makes a smoother oatmeal)**
>
> **2 tablespoons raisins**
>
> **1 tablespoon walnut pieces (or other nuts, as desired)**
>
> **1-2 teaspoons honey or brown sugar**

METHOD

You can cook oatmeal and other whole grains in the microwave or on the stovetop.

Microwave directions: If you choose to microwave, place all ingredients for one serving into each of two bowls large enough to hold the expanding grain. Add water to cover the oatmeal or other grain in each bowl, loosely covering bowls with a paper towel or wax paper, and microwave on high for 1-3 minutes, depending on the grain.

Stovetop directions: If you prefer to cook the oatmeal or other grain on the stovetop, place all ingredients for two servings in a small, uncovered saucepan. Bring to a rolling boil. Immediately turn heat off, leaving the saucepan on the burner, and cover with a lid, checking in the first minute to be sure the oatmeal or grain doesn't boil over. Leave covered for 5 minutes, and then pour into bowls. (Some grains require longer cooking times. Check package.)

Serve with low-fat or skim milk, fat-free half-and-half, or "milk" of your choice and 1 to 2 teaspoons honey or brown sugar.

Serve breakfast with a glass of milk, low-fat or skim, or "milk" of your choice, coffee or tea, and if desired with a sweetener, non-fat half-and-half cream, and fruit such as unsweetened applesauce or cut navel oranges.

Unsweetened Applesauce
Serves 2-4

INGREDIENTS

1 medium jar unsweetened applesauce

½ teaspoon ground cinnamon, optional

METHOD

1. Spoon about ½ cup unsweetened applesauce into each of two small bowls. Sprinkle with ground cinnamon, if using.

2. Serve with rest of breakfast.

Navel Orange
Serves 2

INGREDIENTS

1 navel orange

METHOD

1. Cut the navel orange lengthwise into 4 equal pieces. Peel off rind. Divide the segments. Serve pieces without the rind on a small plate.

MAIN MEAL

Turnip or Mustard Greens

The easiest way to cook this traditional dish is to use pre-washed, chopped greens, canned, or frozen.

Serves 4-6

INGREDIENTS

- **1 large package pre-washed and chopped fresh turnip or mustard greens (available in some produce departments), 2 packages of drained frozen greens, or 2 drained 14.5-ounce cans turnip or mustard greens. Keep the added salt or sugar to a minimum. You can also use 1 head of fresh greens. See above with the Main Meal Menu for directions for cooking these fresh greens.**

- **1 tablespoon extra virgin olive oil or canola oil**

- **1 teaspoon powdered garlic or dried minced garlic or 1 clove garlic, peeled and chopped**

- **1 cup fat-free, low-salt chicken or vegetable broth in a can or carton, or 1 cube of low-salt bouillon**

- **1-2 teaspoons Worcestershire sauce**

- **1-3 drops Tabasco, Texas Pete, or other hot sauce, to taste**

METHOD

1. Add fresh pre-washed packaged, frozen, or canned greens to a large pot or saucepan. If using fresh pre-washed greens, push them down gradually as they cook.

2. While the greens are cooking down, add all other ingredients to the pot or saucepan. Cook over low heat until tender.

3. Remove the greens from the pot or saucepan and reserve the liquid, known as 'pot liquor.' This can be used for dipping cornbread, adding to other cooking vegetables, or even for drinking.

4. Leftover greens can be kept in a container in the refrigerator or frozen until ready to use later.

Black-Eyed Peas
Serves 2-4

INGREDIENTS

1 14-ounce-can black-eyed peas; 1 package frozen black-eyed peas; or 1½ cups cooked and drained dried black-eyed peas, from 16-ounce package, recipe page 225. Be sure there is no added salt or sugar to the canned or frozen black-eyed peas. Sometimes you can find hulled, fresh black-eyed peas in the produce department or at farmers markets.

1 teaspoon extra virgin olive oil or canola oil

½ teaspoon garlic powder, dried minced garlic, or 1 clove garlic, peeled and chopped

2 teaspoons dried onion flakes; dried minced onion or powder; or ½ cup fresh onion, chopped,

1 14-ounce can diced tomatoes, any flavor

⅓ cup beef, chicken, or vegetable broth, low-salt and reduced-fat, from a can or carton, or 1 cube of low-salt bouillon

METHOD

1. Heat oil over medium heat in a large saucepan. If using fresh black-eyed peas, add garlic and onions. Sauté till onions are tender. Add canned diced tomatoes. At this time, add garlic powder or minced dried garlic and onion flakes, powder, or dried minced onion.

2. Add rinsed and drained canned black-eyed peas, frozen black-eyed peas, fresh packaged black-eyed peas, or cooked dried black-eyed peas.

3. Add broth or water to cover about 1 inch above the black-eyed peas. Simmer covered for about an hour. Add liquid as the black-eyed peas are cooking as necessary.

Freeze leftover cooked black-eyed peas for future main meals.

Basic Brown Rice Recipe

If you use pre-cooked packaged or frozen brown rice, be sure there is little added salt or sugar. To prepare, follow package directions.

This is a simple, foolproof method that can be used for most rice recipes. And it is cheaper than prepared rice. It costs about 18 cents a serving. Serves 4

For your convenience this is a repeat recipe.

INGREDIENTS

1 cup long-grain brown rice

1½-2 cups water or broth or mixture of the two (Less water makes a drier rice.)

METHOD

1. Add brown rice to medium sized saucepan with water, broth, or mixture of the two

2. Bring to a full boil. Immediately turn down heat to a simmer and cover saucepan. Check two or three times in the first minutes to make sure the water is not boiling over.

3. Set timer to 50 to 55 minutes and only lift lid when the time is up. Check whether the rice has absorbed all the water and that the rice is fluffy. If all the water is not yet absorbed, cover and continue cooking over very low heat. Check every 10 minutes until the rice is done and the water is absorbed.

4. Leftover brown rice can be stored in resealable plastic bags or a covered container in the refrigerator or frozen for future use. It can be reheated in the microwave in loosely covered containers for 1 to 2 minutes.

Cornbread

"Leftover cornbread can be toasted and enjoyed with breakfast and soups." Carol Cantrell

Cornbread mix: You can easily make cornbread from a mix that only requires egg, milk or buttermilk, and oil. If you use a mix, check to be sure it does not have large amounts of sugar. (Many mixes use too much sugar so the "cornbread" is really a cake.) Once you find a healthy cornbread mix, use it whenever you make cornbread.

Cornbread from scratch: This recipe is a Southern classic—a quick and easy recipe. Once you make it this way, you'll do it again and again instead of using a mix. Homemade cornbread has less salt and sugar than a mix. (Look for stone ground or whole grain corn meal.)

Serves 6-8

INGREDIENTS

> **1 cup yellow or white cornmeal, stone ground or whole grain is preferred**
>
> **1 cup whole wheat flour**
>
> **1 teaspoon sugar**
>
> **1 teaspoon baking powder**
>
> **½ teaspoon baking soda, if using buttermilk**
>
> **½ teaspoon salt or to taste, keeping salt to a minimum**
>
> **1 egg**
>
> **1¼ cups low-fat buttermilk, or milk, skim or low-fat, or "milk" of your choice. Add liquid as necessary to make pour-able batter. If not using buttermilk, omit the baking soda.**
>
> **2 tablespoons extra virgin olive oil or canola oil**

METHOD

1. Preheat oven to 425 degrees. Place an 8-inch cast iron skillet in the oven with about 1 tablespoon oil in the bottom. Or oil an 8-inch square baking pan or dish. With the baking pan or

dish you may use nonstick cooking spray. The cast iron gives a crisper crust.

2. In a large bowl, mix together cornmeal, flour, baking powder, baking soda (if using with buttermilk), and salt.

3. Add egg, buttermilk or milk, and oil and stir till just combined.

4. Pour batter into sizzling hot, oiled skillet or baking pan, and then bake 20 to 25 minutes. The cornbread is done when lightly golden, pulls away from skillet or pan, and a knife comes out clean when inserted. Cool for a few minutes and then carefully invert onto a plate.

5. Cut into about 8 wedges or pieces and then serve while still warm with your main meal. At breakfast, warmed cornbread is good spread with honey or jam, or dipped in the yolk of fried eggs.

6. Save leftover cornbread in the refrigerator or freezer.

7. You can add as you are mixing to your cornbread: 1 teaspoon cumin powder; 1 teaspoon chili powder; ½ to 1 cup corn kernels either frozen, canned and drained or fresh corn; 1 tablespoon bacon bits; ½ to 1 cup shredded Monterey jack cheese or similar cheese; 1 4-ounce can minced green chili; or other combinations or items that will enhance the cornbread's flavor.

Recipe tested by Carol Cantrell

Baked Pears

"It's a great recipe." Emma Allan

Serves 2

INGREDIENTS

1 pear, Anjou or other firm pear, 1 package frozen sliced pears, or 1 14.5-ounce can of sliced pears packed in fruit juice

2 teaspoons honey

½ teaspoon ground cinnamon, optional

2 tablespoons low-fat or no-fat vanilla or Greek yogurt, vanilla ice milk, or vanilla frozen yogurt

METHOD

1. Preheat oven to 375 degrees. Mix honey with ground cinnamon, if using, and spread in the bottom of a small baking pan or dish.

2. If using a fresh pear, wash, halve, and remove core and seeds. You may leave the peel on if you wish. Place pears cut side down in prepared pan or dish. If using canned or frozen pears, spread drained pears across bottom of pan or dish, reserving liquid.

3. Place pan in oven and bake about 10 to 15 minutes. Do not let pears overcook and become mushy.

4. Remove from oven and place about ½ the baked pears with some honey from bottom of baking pan in each individual serving dish. Top each with 1 tablespoon plain or frozen yogurt.

Recipe tested by Emma Allan

LIGHT MEAL

Easy Basic Soup

"This soup is NOT HARD TO MAKE!!!. Don't let the recipe fool you. There's nothing to it." Carol Cantrell

Very easy to make and a good last minute dish. You can adjust this soup to what you have on hand at the moment.

Serves 4-6

INGREDIENTS

1 tablespoon extra virgin olive oil or canola oil

If using fresh ingredients:

½ onion, chopped

1 clove garlic, peeled and chopped

½ cup bell pepper, green, yellow, or red, chopped, optional

If using dried and jarred ingredients:

1-2 teaspoons each powdered or minced dried onion and garlic

1 16-ounce jar of salsa (instead of the chopped bell pepper—beware of high salt content)

2 cups pre-washed packaged shredded or chopped vegetables such as carrots, beans, broccoli, cauliflower, cabbage, and more. If using canned or frozen, use low-salt and no-fat. Or use the vegetables you have on hand.

1 14.5-ounce can tomatoes, diced, any flavor

1 can beans, white, black, red, or your choice, rinsed and drained to get rid of the extra salt, 1 cup cooked dried beans from a 16-ounce package, recipe page 226, or 1 package frozen beans

137

> **2 cups canned or boxed broth, beef, chicken, or vegetable, low-salt and reduced-fat. Reserve remaining broth for future use.**
>
> **About 1 cup water or more to mix with the broth and cover vegetables**

If you use meat:

> **1 cup cooked chicken, beef, ham, or pork, chopped or diced, to put in the broth/water to add flavor. You can use any leftover meat for this soup, or just the beans if you prefer.**

> **½ cup small uncooked whole grain, such as pasta, brown rice, barley, or other grain**

> **2 teaspoons dried herbs such as thyme, oregano, basil**

Salt and pepper to taste, if needed

METHOD

1. Heat oil in bottom of medium or large saucepan.
2. Wash, seed, and remove pith of a bell pepper, chop the onion and garlic if using fresh. Add fresh chopped onion and garlic to the oil in the saucepan and sauté for about 5 minutes or less. Add bell pepper and sauté until the bell pepper begins to turn limp.
3. If using meat, add to the pan and sauté until turning brown.
4. Add other selected vegetables and canned diced tomatoes to the saucepan. Stir and sauté for about 5 minutes.
5. If using dried onion and garlic as well as jarred salsa, first add the jar of salsa to the saucepan. Then add powdered or dried onion and garlic.
6. Add beans and stir again. Mix well.
7. Add broth and water to cover the ingredients. Add uncooked grains and stir. (Add cooked grains in the last 20 minutes of cooking.) Bring to a full, rolling boil and then immediately turn down heat so soup simmers, covered, for about 1 to 2 hours.

8. In the last 30 minutes, add selected herbs, salt, and pepper to taste. Check the grains for doneness. Taste soup and adjust seasonings as necessary.

9. Serve in bowls with heated cornbread or other whole grain bread on the side. Reserve leftover soup for future use.

Recipe tested by Carol Cantrell

Cornbread

Select 2 to 4 pieces of leftover cornbread from freezer or refrigerator. Or make fresh cornbread from Main Meal recipe, page 134.

SNACKS

Banana, Peanut Butter, and Whole Grain Bread or Crackers

Serves 2

INGREDIENTS

1 piece of whole grain bread or 2 small crackers

1 tablespoon natural peanut butter with no added salt, sugar, or fat

1 small ripe banana

METHOD

1. Spread peanut butter evenly on bread or crackers. Slice banana and place slices on bread or crackers with peanut butter.

2. Divide bread, if using, into two pieces and serve prepared bread or crackers with glasses of milk, low-fat or skim, or "milk" of your choice.

Apple and Cheese
Serves 2

INGREDIENTS

1 whole apple

2 slices reduced-fat cheese such as part-skim Mozzarella

METHOD

1. Thoroughly wash apple. Cut into quarters and remove core, seeds, and peel. (Preparing the apple is easier in this order.)

2. Serve with mozzarella and beverage of your choice. (See Chapter 7, "Drink Up! What You Drink Is Important," pages 40-44.)

Day 2 Menus

BREAKFAST

- Eggs, Over Light
- Frozen Whole Grain Waffles with Sautéed Apple Slices with Maple Syrup or Honey
- Low-Fat or Skim Milk or "Milk" of Your Choice
- Coffee or Tea

MAIN MEAL

- Satisfying Quick Chili
- Sour Cream, Low-Fat or Fat-Free
- Brown Rice, or Other Whole Grain
- Salad with Cherry Tomatoes and Salad Dressing
- Cornbread or Sliced Whole Wheat Baguette
- Vanilla Yogurt with Graham Cracker

LIGHT MEAL

- Simple and Easy Split Pea Soup
- Whole Wheat Crackers, Cornbread, or Baguette

SNACKS

- Walnut and Raisins, Dried Cranberries, or other Dried Fruit
- Yogurt with Banana

Day 2 Recipes
BREAKFAST

Eggs over Light

Eggs prepared this way go well with waffles. You can cook the eggs as the apple slices are cooking and frozen waffles are heating.

Serves 2

INGREDIENTS

2 teaspoons extra virgin olive oil or canola oil

2 large eggs

METHOD

1. Place oil in small frying pan and heat on medium low heat. Break eggs, one at a time, into a small bowl.

2. Slide one egg into the heated frying pan and cook on one side until the white firms, about 4-5 minutes. When the white is beginning to firm, turn the egg over and let cook for 30 seconds to 1 minute.

3. Remove from pan to serving plate. Repeat with the other egg. Keep warm.

Frozen Whole Grain Waffles with Sautéed Apple Slices
Serves 2

INGREDIENTS

2-4 frozen whole grain waffles, with little or no added sugar, salt, or fats

1 apple, such as gala, delicious, or other sweet apple

1 teaspoon butter and 1 teaspoon extra virgin olive oil or canola oil

2-4 teaspoons maple syrup or honey

METHOD

1. Place 2 to 4 whole-grain waffles in toaster set to warm or toast. Wait until the last minute before heating and serving.

2. Wash and cut apple into quarters, and then core and seed. Peel, if desired. Then cut the quartered and cored apple pieces into thin slices. This task is much easier in this order.

3. On medium heat, melt butter with oil in medium non-stick skillet. When butter is melted, add apple slices and cook on one side for about 3 to 4 minutes till beginning to brown. Turn and repeat.

4. Sautéed apple slices make a healthy topping for cooked cereals, desserts, chicken, pork chops, and other dishes.

5. Place warmed or toasted waffles on plates with sautéed apples on top.

6. Put eggs on the same plate with the waffles. Put maple syrup or honey on the table. Serve with glass of low-fat or skim milk or "milk" of your choice, and coffee or tea with sugar and fat-free half-and-half cream on the side to use as desired.

MAIN MEAL

Satisfying Quick Chili with Sour Cream

"This chili is really tasty, and after a day in the refrigerator, it is delicious." Ruth Porter

Perfect for cold evenings and when you're out of energy and time. There'll be leftovers to save for another night. (I love leftovers!) Though the ingredient list looks long, this is extremely easy to make. And so good!

Serves 4-6

INGREDIENTS

1 tablespoon extra virgin olive oil or canola oil

½ pound 93 to 96% lean ground beef, ground chicken breast, or other lean meat pieces (You can skip the meat addition entirely and just add beans for the protein.)

1 cup pre-washed packaged bell pepper or ½ bell pepper, pith removed, seeded, and chopped

3 teaspoons powdered or minced dried onion or ½ onion, chopped

1½ teaspoons powdered or minced dried garlic or 2 cloves fresh garlic, peeled and chopped

2 14.5-ounce cans diced tomatoes, any flavor

1 14.5-ounce can beans—black or pinto are good with chili, or beans of your choice, rinsed and drained to remove excess salt, or 1-1 ½ cups precooked dried beans from a 16-ounce package, recipe page 225

2 teaspoons dried cilantro or 1 bunch fresh cilantro, chopped, optional

1 tablespoon ground cumin seed (This spice is often used in Mexican or Spanish dishes.)

About 1 teaspoon each dried herbs such as oregano and basil, or to taste

1-3 teaspoons chili powder (start with lower amount and adjust to taste)

1 small can green chili peppers, diced, mild or hot, optional

1 small jar salsa, optional (Salsa adds Mexican flavor to this easy chili.)

1 teaspoon salt, if needed

2-4 teaspoons cornmeal, if necessary, to thicken

1½ tablespoons extra dark cocoa, optional (This is a Mexican-style addition to chili and makes it delicious.)

METHOD

1. Brown meat, if using, in oil in a medium-sized saucepan.

2. Add to the pot or saucepan: Chopped bell pepper, fresh onion, and fresh garlic, if using. Cook on low until vegetables are tender.

3. Add chopped, canned tomatoes, beans, cilantro, if using, ground cumin seed, other herbs, chili powder, canned diced chili peppers, salsa, and powdered or minced dried garlic and onion, if using. Stir to mix well.

4. Adjust seasonings as needed. If the chili needs thickening as it cooks, add 1 to 2 teaspoons cornmeal at a time, up to 4 teaspoons. After each addition, allow the chili to simmer for about 5 minutes before adding more. As the chili stands after cooking, it will thicken.

5. Cook covered over very low heat for 2 to 3 hours. Serve over rice or other grain. The taste of this chili improves the next day.

6. Place in serving-size containers and freeze leftover chili for future use.

Recipe tested by Ruth Porter

Brown Rice

Reheat in a microwave on high two portions of refrigerated or frozen brown rice in a loosely covered bowl for 1 to 1½ minutes. If you make Brown Rice from scratch, use the recipe, page 80, or make it from frozen or boxed pre-cooked.

Salad with Cherry Tomatoes and Salad Dressing
This salad depends on what you have on hand and your creativity.
Serves 2

INGREDIENTS

2 cups pre-washed packaged Romaine lettuce or 3-4 cups washed and drained torn Romaine lettuce leaves, or lettuce of your choice

3-4 washed cherry or grape tomatoes, if available, halved

2 teaspoons powdered or dried minced onion or ¼-½ cup onion, your choice, thinly sliced

1 tablespoon salad dressing, either bottle low-fat, low-salt, such as Caesar or Italian, or Homemade, recipe page 83

Optional: You can add any number of vegetables to this salad, including chopped carrots, broccoli, cauliflower, bell pepper, cabbage, and more. Many of these vegetables are available in pre-washed packaged shredded or chopped. You can also add chopped nuts such as almonds, pecans, or walnuts and halved grapes or other fruits.

METHOD

1. Tear or cut lettuce into pieces. Place in medium-sized bowl.
2. Add halved tomatoes, thinly sliced onion, and other optional vegetables, nuts, or fruit.
3. Add about 1 tablespoon salad dressing to the salad and toss with large spoons.

Whole Wheat Baguette

Buy 1 whole wheat baguette. Slice diagonally across the long part into 2-to-3-inch slices. Place all unused slices in freezer bag and freeze for future use.

Warm, not toast, 2 to 4 slices baguette in a toaster oven and serve with extra virgin olive oil or canola oil for dipping or to spread on top. You can solidify olive oil by placing in a wide-mouth jar or container and refrigerating until it hardens.

Cornbread

Take pieces from freezer if available. These were made from the cornbread recipe, page 134.

LIGHT MEAL

Simple and Easy Split Pea Soup
Serves 4-6

INGREDIENTS

1 16-ounce package dried split peas

1 tablespoon extra virgin olive oil or canola oil

2 teaspoons onion powder; dried minced onion; or ½ cup onion, chopped

4-6 baby carrots, sliced; 1 whole carrot, washed, scraped and sliced; or ½ cup shredded pre-washed, packaged carrots, optional

1 cup bell pepper from pre-washed packaged bell pepper or fresh, washed, halved, pith removed, seeded, and chopped, optional

1-2 teaspoons dried thyme, sage, basil, or other dried herb of your choice (You can add 1-2 teaspoons curry powder for an Asian taste.)

1 can or carton beef, chicken, or vegetarian broth plus enough water to cover dried split peas by about 1 inch

Salt and pepper to taste

METHOD

1. Pour dried split peas into a colander or sieve. Remove stones or misshapen peas from batch. Rinse thoroughly, allowing the water to run through the colander for a minute or so.

4. Heat oil in a large pot or saucepan. Sauté over medium-low heat the onion, carrots, and bell pepper till soft and starting to brown, about 10 minutes.

5. At this time, add rinsed split peas and stir. Add powdered or dried minced onion, if using; broth; and water to cover about 1 inch. Increase heat to high and bring to a full boil.

6. Lower heat immediately to low until the mixture comes to a simmer, cover, and let cook for about 20 to 30 minutes or more. The peas should be tender but not mushy.

7. Near the end of the cooking time add fresh or dried thyme, sage, basil, or other herbs or curry. (If you like softer peas, continue cooking until they are the consistency you prefer.)

8. Serve in bowls with whole wheat crackers on the side, re-heated cornbread, or sliced baguette.

9. Freeze or refrigerate leftover soup for future use.

SNACKS

Walnuts and Raisins, Dried Cranberries, or Other Dried Fruit
Serves 2 or more

INGREDIENTS

1 cup roasted walnut pieces, or nut of your choice (Unroasted or raw nuts are usually available in the produce section of the grocery store. One package may seem expensive but it lasts for a long time.)

1 cup dried raisins, dried cranberries, or chopped dried fruit of your choice

METHOD

1. Roast walnut pieces by spreading all the raw nuts that are in a package (probably more than 1 cup), unsalted, on a rimmed cookie sheet. Bake in a 350-degree oven for 8 to 9 minutes, being sure they don't overcook. Remove from the oven and allow to cool. Store any unused walnuts in a baggie or jar for future use. By roasting all the nuts in the package at one time, you save time, energy, and money.

2. Combine 1 cup roasted walnut pieces and 1 cup raisins or other dried fruit in a plastic container for easy access. Eat small amounts from the container and keep remainders for future use.

Yogurt with Bananas

Serves 2

INGREDIENTS

¾ cup plain yogurt or Greek yogurt, low-fat or fat-free

1 ripe banana

2 teaspoons honey

METHOD

1. Divide yogurt into two small bowls. Cut banana into slices crosswise, placing ½ the sliced banana into each bowl. Add honey. Stir and serve.

Day 3 Menus

`SUPER EASY`

BREAKFAST

➤ Two Eggs, Scrambled

➤ Two Slices Toasted Whole Wheat Bread with Soft-Tub Margarine[1] and Low-Sugar Preserves or Jam or Honey

➤ Navel Orange

➤ Skim or Low-Fat Milk or "Milk" of Your Choice

➤ Coffee or Tea

> [1]Use soft-tub margarine that contains no animal fat or hydrogenated fat. There are many brands. Read the Nutrition Facts label before choosing.

`SUPER EASY`

MAIN MEAL

➤ Simple Everyday Pork Chops

➤ Cuban-Style Black Beans and Brown Rice

➤ Simple Salad with Tomatoes and Vegetables

➤ Pumpkin Pudding with Sautéed Apple Slices

`SUPER EASY`

LIGHT MEAL

➤ Cheese Melt with Tomato Slice on Whole Wheat Bread

`SUPER EASY`

SNACKS

➤ Banana with Peanut Butter

➤ Plain Instant Oatmeal with Nuts and Applesauce

Day 3 Recipes
BREAKFAST

Two Eggs, Scrambled, with Whole Wheat Bread,
Soft-Tub Margarine, and Low-Sugar Preserves,
Jam, or Honey with a Navel Orange
Serves 2

INGREDIENTS

> **2 whole wheat bread slices or whole grain bread of your choice**
>
> **2 teaspoons soft-tub margarine**
>
> **2 teaspoons extra virgin olive oil or canola oil**
>
> **2 eggs, broken into a small bowl**
>
> **1 teaspoon water**
>
> **1 navel orange, quartered**
>
> **2 teaspoons low-sugar preserves, jam, or honey**
>
> **2 glasses skim or low-fat milk or "milk" of your choice, or water**
>
> **Coffee or tea**

METHOD

1. Begin toasting the bread and quartering the navel orange before you scramble the eggs so they will all be ready at about the same time.

2. Add the oil to a small non-stick skillet over medium-low heat. Break two eggs into a small bowl and beat with a fork or spoon. Add 1 teaspoon water to the beaten eggs.

3. When the oil in the frying pan is heated, pour the eggs into heated pan and with a spatula, turn the outsides of the cooking eggs into the center. Continue until the eggs are at your preferred firmness. Remove from the pan and place on the plates. Keep warm.

4. Add the quartered and peeled navel orange segments to the plates along with the toasted whole wheat or whole grain bread. Place soft-tub margarine and jam or honey on the table. Spread 1 teaspoon margarine on each slice of toast as needed.

5. Serve skim or low-fat milk or "milk" of your choice, or water and coffee or tea with little or no added sugar or fat-free half-and-half cream.

MAIN MEAL

Simple Everyday Pork Chops

Many pork chops these days are a lean, white meat. Buy your pork chops with very little fat marbling, either sliced thinly or thickly, usually without a bone. Before you cook, trim off the fat that may be bordering the chop.

Serves 2

INGREDIENTS

2 teaspoons extra virgin olive oil or canola oil

2 pork chops with little fat marbling, with or without the bone

1 teaspoon dried sage, optional

Salt and pepper to taste

METHOD

1. Rub the sage, if using, into the pork chop before cooking. Let it sit while the oil heats in the skillet.

2. Add oil to a medium to large nonstick skillet. Heat on medium-high. When hot, add the prepared pork chops to the pan and cook on one side for 1 to 2 minutes for a thinly sliced pork chop and for 2 to 4 minutes for a thick cut. While cooking, salt and pepper the pork chops to taste, using a minimum salt.

3. Turn and cook on the other side for about 2 to 4 minutes depending on the thickness of the chop. The pork chop is done when the meat turns a pale pink or white. Salt and pepper a final time to taste.

4. Remove from the skillet to plates. Serve.

Cuban-Style Black Beans and Brown Rice

"This is delicious." Ruth Porter

In South Florida, this dish is readily found. It's extremely easy to make and offers protein, fiber, and lots of flavor. You can serve this as a side dish or as a meal in itself with a salad. The Cubans use white rice, but we're going to serve it the healthy way with brown rice.

Serves 4-6

INGREDIENTS

> 1 tablespoon extra virgin olive oil or canola oil
>
> 1 teaspoon powdered or dried minced onion or 1 cup onion, chopped
>
> 1 cup pre-washed packaged bell pepper, or 1 cup fresh bell pepper, pith removed, seeded, and chopped
>
> 3 teaspoons powdered or dried minced garlic or 5 cloves garlic, peeled and chopped
>
> Pinch of chili powder, optional
>
> 1 14.5-ounce can diced tomatoes, your choice of flavor
>
> 2 15-ounce cans black beans, rinsed and drained
>
> 1 teaspoon dried cilantro or ½ bunch fresh cilantro, optional
>
> Salt and pepper to taste
>
> 1 lime, cut into wedges for garnish, optional

METHOD

1. Heat large skillet over medium high heat. When skillet is hot, add oil.

2. Sauté fresh onion, if using, for about 1 minute, or until translucent but not brown. Add the fresh bell pepper, fresh garlic, and chili powder, if using. Continue to sauté until bell pepper becomes tender.

3. Reduce heat to low and add diced tomatoes and cilantro, if using.

4. At this time add the powdered or dried minced onion and garlic. Stir. Simmer, uncovered, about 15 minutes.

5. Add rinsed and drained black beans and simmer for another 10 minutes. Add salt and pepper to taste, keeping it to a minimum.

6. Serve with brown rice (recipe page 80) and lime wedges on the side.

Recipe tested by Ruth Porter

Pumpkin Pudding

"I liked this! Especially with the ginger." Angela Eberts

Serves 8-10

INGREDIENTS

2 eggs

1 12-ounce can evaporated skim milk

1 15-ounce-can pumpkin puree with no additives

½ cup packed brown sugar or dark molasses or honey or combination of sweets that will equal ½ cup, adjust to taste

¼ teaspoon salt

1 teaspoon ground cinnamon

½ teaspoon ground ginger, optional

2 teaspoons vanilla

METHOD

1. Preheat oven to 425 degrees. In a medium-sized bowl, beat the eggs and evaporated milk with a fork until combined. Add all the other ingredients and stir well until smooth.

2. Pour mixture into an oiled 10-inch pie plate, baking dish, or 8 to 10 individual custard cups. Place filled container(s) on a rimmed cookie sheet that has been covered with aluminum foil and bake at 425 degrees for 20 minutes. Then lower heat to 350 degrees and bake for another 30 to 40 minutes. The custard cups will take 20 to 30 minutes.

3. Check after 20 minutes. A knife inserted into the center should come out clean. Serve ½ cup servings as is or top with sautéed apple slices.

Recipe tested by Angela Eberts

Sautéed Apple Slices

These sautéed apples are a topping that can substitute for high-fat, high-calorie, and high-sugar ice cream or whipped cream toppings over desserts, waffles, cereal, and other dishes that need sweets. See page 141.

Serves 2-4

INGREDIENTS

1 apple such as gala, delicious, or other sweet apple

1 tablespoon extra virgin olive oil or canola oil

1 teaspoon sweet butter

METHOD

1. Wash apple thoroughly and cut into quarters, then core and seed. Peel, if desired. Cut the quartered and cored apple pieces into thin slices. This task is much easier in this order.

2. On medium heat, melt butter with oil in medium non-stick skillet. When butter is melted, add apple slices and cook on one side for about 3 to 4 minutes till they are beginning to brown. Turn and repeat.

3. Serve over Pumpkin Pudding, waffles, pie, or other dishes you wish to sweeten.

SNACKS

Banana with Peanut Butter

If you're taking this to work, place the banana with peanut butter in a covered plastic container. When serving at work or at home, spread small amounts of softened peanut butter on each piece of the banana. Eat it with a fork or spoon. You may spread the peanut butter on crackers and then top with the sliced banana, if desired.

You can use other nut butters, such as almond or cashew, both are more expensive than peanut butter. (Nut butters are soft at room temperature.)

Plain Instant Oatmeal with Nuts

Use one package of plain instant oatmeal for each serving and, following package directions, add water to the oatmeal in bowls large enough for the oatmeal to expand. Heat in a microwave according to package directions. When serving, add ¼ cup nuts such as chopped walnuts or almonds and 1 tablespoon unsweetened applesauce.

Day 4 Menus

SUPER EASY

BREAKFAST

➤ Whole Grain Bagel with Low-Fat Cream Cheese, Neufchatel, or Greek Yogurt

➤ Low-Sugar Preserves, Jam, or Honey

➤ Black Seedless Grapes or Other Kinds of Grapes

➤ Low-Fat or Skim Milk or "Milk," or Water

➤ Coffee or Tea

SUPER EASY:

MAIN MEAL

➤ Hamburgers on Whole-Grain Buns with Lettuce, Onion, and Tomatoes

➤ Condiments of Choice

➤ Figs or Plums with Greek Yogurt and Almonds

> Note: Lean ground beef contains 3 grams saturated fats and 131 calories in a 3-ounce serving. Whereas 4 ounces of lean ground turkey has 2 grams saturated fats and 160 calories. The 2010 Dietary Guidelines for Americans, updated in March 2012, suggest that you consume less than 10 percent of your calories from saturated fats, or less than 200 calories a day based on a 2000-calorie diet.

SUPER EASY

LIGHT MEAL

➤ Vegetable Salad with Reduced-Fat Cheese Slices with Whole Wheat Pita

➤ Applesauce with Cinnamon

SUPER EASY:

SNACKS

➤ Apple with Cheese

➤ Cottage Cheese or Greek Yogurt and Fruit

Day 4 Recipes
BREAKFAST

Whole Grain Bagel with Low-Fat or Fat-Free Cream Cheese, Neufchatel, or Greek Yogurt
Serves 2

INGREDIENTS

> 2 tablespoons low-fat or fat-free cream cheese, Neufchatel, or Greek yogurt
>
> 2 small whole grain bagels or 1 large whole grain bagel, sliced
>
> 2 teaspoons low-sugar preserves, jam, or honey
>
> 1-2 cups black seedless grapes or grapes of your choice

METHOD

1. Bring cream cheese or Neufchatel, if serving, to room temperature and place 1 tablespoon cream cheese, Neufchatel, or Greek yogurt on each of two plates along with 1 teaspoon low-sugar jam or honey.

2. Slice bagels in half and place cut-side up on a toaster oven tray. Toast until light brown.

3. Place ½ to 1 cup black seedless grapes or grapes of your choice into each of 2 small bowls. Serve with low-fat or skim milk or water, and coffee or tea with a minimum of fat-free half-and-half cream or sugar.

MAIN MEAL

Hamburgers on Whole Grain Buns with Lettuce, Onion, and Tomatoes
Serves 2

INGREDIENTS

1 teaspoon powdered or dried minced garlic or 1 clove garlic, peeled and chopped

1 teaspoon each oregano and basil, dried

½ pound 93-96% lean ground beef or low-fat lean ground turkey breast, mixed half and half with the beef, or entirely ground turkey

½ cup dry regular or quick cooking oatmeal

1 egg

2 tablespoons extra virgin olive oil or canola oil

2 whole grain buns, sliced

2 large lettuce leaves

2 slices onion

2 slices tomato, if available

½ teaspoon each of condiments, such as mustard, lite mayonnaise, and ketchup, your choice

METHOD

1. Add garlic, herbs, oatmeal, egg to ground beef, or a mix of the ground beef and ground turkey, or the ground turkey. If using only the turkey, add 1 tablespoon oil.

2. Mix thoroughly with a large spoon or your hands. Shape the ground meat into 2 patties.

3. Place 1 tablespoon oil in medium size non-stick skillet and heat on medium till shimmering, about 5 minutes. Add patties and cook till brown on one side, about 3 minutes, and turn. Lower heat to medium low and cook for another 5 to 7 minutes.

4. Meanwhile, toast buns with the cut side up until they are light brown. Place on a plate with lettuce, tomato, and onion.

5. When the hamburger patties are done, place them on the open toasted buns and serve with condiments on the side.

6. Use very little of the condiments since they are high in salt, fat, and sugar. A little will go a long way.

Figs or Plums with Greek Yogurt and Almonds
Serves 2

INGREDIENTS

**1 can of figs with no added sugar or 2 ripe figs
(Canned or fresh plums may be substituted.)**

½ cup low-fat or fat-free Greek yogurt

2 teaspoons honey, or to taste

¼ cup slivered, roasted almonds

METHOD

1. To make roasted almonds: (Raw nuts are available in the produce section of the grocery store. The amount of nuts in these packages will last a long time.) Prepare more than you will use for this recipe and reserve the remainder in a closed plastic container or jar for future use. These roasted nuts are good in salads, soups, or desserts.

2. Preheat oven to 350 degrees. Spread a medium or large size bag of slivered almonds on a rimmed cookie sheet and place in the pre-heated oven. Set timer for 9 minutes, being careful not to leave almonds in the heat too long since they will burn. After 8 or 9 minutes, remove from the oven and cool. Store remaining nuts in a plastic container or jar with lids for future use.

3. Remove ¼ cup almonds for this recipe. Cut the figs or plums in half and place on dessert plates. Top each half with ¼ cup Greek yogurt and sprinkle with the roasted almonds.

LIGHT MEAL

Vegetable Salad with Reduced-Fat Cheese Slices with Whole Wheat Pita

Serves 2

INGREDIENTS

1½ to 2 cups pre-washed packaged cut vegetables, such as lettuce, carrots, celery, broccoli, cauliflower, and cabbage, or prepare your own choice of vegetables

2 slices reduced-fat cheese, such as Swiss, cheddar, Monterey jack, part-skim mozzarella, or your choice, cut into small pieces

1 tablespoon bottled salad dressing, low-fat and low-salt, such as Italian or Caesar, or Homemade Salad Dressing, recipe page 83

Salt and pepper to taste

METHOD

Place all ingredients in a bowl. Toss until well mixed. Taste and adjust amount of salad dressing and salt and pepper. Serve.

Whole Wheat Pita

Place 1 whole wheat pita in a toaster oven on warm for 5 minutes. Divide into 4 to 6 wedges. Serve 1 to 2 wedges on each plate with the salad, vegetables, and cheese.

Applesauce with Cinnamon

Serves 2 to 4

INGREDIENTS

1 small jar unsweetened natural applesauce

½ teaspoon lemon juice from fresh lemon or from bottled pure lemon juice, optional

½ teaspoon ground cinnamon, optional

1 teaspoon sugar or honey, if necessary

METHOD

1. Buy 1 small jar of natural, unsweetened applesauce. Pour contents into a small bowl and add the lemon juice and cinnamon, if using. Serve ½ cup in each of two bowls, adding ½ teaspoon sugar or honey if desired.

2. Return prepared applesauce to the jar and place in the refrigerator for future use.

SNACKS

Apple with Cheese

Serves 2

INGREDIENTS

½ apple, such as gala, delicious, Macintosh, or your choice

1 slice reduced-fat cheese, such as mozzarella or Swiss

METHOD

Slice apple into quarters, core, seed, and peel, if desired. (Reserve the other half in a covered container in the refrigerator for future use.) Serve slices with reduced-fat cheese.

Cottage Cheese or Greek Yogurt and Fruit

Serves 2

INGREDIENTS

1 cup low-fat or fat-free cottage cheese or Greek yogurt

1 cup fresh fruit, such as banana, apple, or grapes, or canned or frozen fruit, your choice. (If using canned, be sure it's packed in fruit juices and contains no added sugar.)

METHOD

Place ½ cup cottage cheese or Greek yogurt into each of 2 bowls. Top with fruit of your choice.

Day 5 Menus

BREAKFAST

➤ Cooked Hot Whole Grain Cereal[1] with Low-Fat or Skim Milk or "Milk," and Fruit and Nuts

➤ Greek Yogurt with Honey

➤ Coffee or Tea

> [1]There are several hot whole grain cereals that are delicious, such as Wheatena, Roman Meal hot cereals, oatmeal, Irish oatmeal, oatmeal bran, and other whole grain hot cereals. You can make it easier for yourself by cooking for 3 to 4 days at a time and saving servings for the following days in plastic containers. Heat loosely covered in a microwave for about 1 to 2 minutes to serve. Make sure the hot cereals are whole grain. To cook follow the package directions.

MAIN MEAL

➤ Quick Lasagna

➤ Simple Salad with Tomatoes, Vegetables, Fruit, and Nuts

➤ Whole Wheat Baguette

➤ Broiled Pineapple Slices

LIGHT MEAL

➤ Toasted Cheese with Tomato Slice

➤ Broccoli Slaw

SNACKS

➤ Granola Bar, High Protein[1]

➤ Hummus and Cut Vegetables (Crudités)

> [1]Look for a high-protein, low-fat, low-sugar snack bar. Be careful. Many snack bars are really candy in disguise.

Day 5 Recipes

BREAKFAST

Cooked Hot Whole Grain Cereal with Low-Fat or Skim Milk or "Milk" of Your Choice, Fruit and Nuts, Greek Yogurt with Honey, Coffee or Tea
Serves 2

INGREDIENTS

- 2 servings from package of whole grain hot cereal, your choice. Selection includes regular, quick, and instant oatmeal; Wheatena, Roman Meal hot cereals, Irish oatmeal, oatmeal bran, and others
- ½ cup raisins or other dried fruit or 1 cup fresh, frozen, or canned fruit such as strawberries, blueberries, peaches, or your choice. Make sure the frozen or canned has no added sugar.
- ½ cup nuts, such as chopped walnuts, pecans, slivered almonds, or your choice
- Low-fat or skim milk, "milk" of your choice, or fat-free half-and-half cream
- 2 teaspoons brown sugar or honey, if necessary

METHOD

1. Follow package directions to cook the cereal of your choice, either in the microwave or on the stovetop. Add dried fruit and nuts before cooking. Add ½ cup fresh, frozen, or canned fruit to each serving after cooking.

2. Serve in two bowls with brown sugar or honey and low-fat, skim milk, or "milk" of your choice, or fat-free half-and-half cream.

3. In another two bowls, add ½ cup low-fat or fat-free Greek yogurt to each. Sweeten each with ½ teaspoon honey. Greek yogurt adds more protein to your breakfast.

4. Serve with coffee or tea, as you wish, with fat-free half-and-half cream or sweetener, as needed.

Main Meal

Quick Lasagna

"This was easy to make and will be especially useful for working families who want a healthy one-dish meal that can be cooked the day or weekend ahead and warmed up quickly for dinner." Angela Eberts

This Quick Lasagna can be made with or without the thawed frozen spinach. The spaghetti sauce can be with or without meat. By using spaghetti sauce in a jar, you are saving a step in the preparation of this dish, and by using dried herbs you can make this dish more quickly. Or you can make your own sauce simply and easily and save leftovers for use in many dishes.

Serves 6-8

INGREDIENTS

2 teaspoons extra virgin olive oil or canola oil

1 package frozen chopped spinach, thawed (if using)

1 small can sliced mushrooms or 1 cup from
1 package sliced mushrooms, optional

1 pound part-skim ricotta or low-fat or fat-free
creamy cottage cheese

2 cups shredded or chopped reduced-fat mozzarella

1 egg

1 teaspoon dried oregano or 2 tablespoons fresh
oregano

1 teaspoon dried basil or 2 tablespoons fresh basil

¼ teaspoon dried nutmeg or ¼ teaspoon freshly
grated nutmeg

Salt and pepper to taste

4 cups of spaghetti sauce in a jar, your choice of
flavors, or from spaghetti sauce recipe, page 228

1 package lasagna noodles, whole wheat, if available
(Save remaining dry noodles for future use.)

½ to ¾ cup water

½ cup Parmesan cheese, grated or shredded

METHOD

1. Thaw spinach, if using. (This will take as much as 3 to 4 hours.) Squeeze out as much moisture from the thawed spinach as possible.

2. Preheat oven to 350 degrees. Lightly oil rectangular baking pan. Use a pan that is approximately 2 inches deep and at least 8 x 10 inches over all.

3. In a small non-stick skillet, sauté in the oil the fresh mushrooms, if using. Cool and set aside.

4. Mix together in a medium-sized bowl, the ricotta or cottage cheese, 1 cup chopped or shredded mozzarella, egg, spinach if using, oregano, basil, nutmeg, salt, and pepper.

5. Place 1 to 2 tablespoons of spaghetti sauce on the bottom of a baking pan. Lay dry noodles on top of the sauce. Cover with half the cheese mixture. Place half the mushrooms, if using, in a layer over the cheese mixture.

6. Repeat with another layer of dry noodles, cheese mixture, and mushrooms, if using. Cover the second layer with the remaining sauce. Sprinkle 1 cup shredded or chopped mozzarella on top.

7. Pour ½ cup water around edges of pan with the uncooked lasagna noodles. (The lasagna noodles will cook as it bakes.) Cover pan tightly with aluminum foil. Carefully place in the middle of the oven and bake at 350 for 1 hour. Remove the foil and top with the Parmesan cheese. Bake for 15 minutes more if necessary or until the liquid has been absorbed.

8. To serve, cut into 3 x 3 inch squares. Refrigerate or freeze leftovers for another meal. This recipe is enough for leftovers for a couple of meals. You can reheat either in the microwave for 1 to 3 minutes or in the oven or toaster oven.

Recipe tested by Angela Eberts

Simple Salad with Tomatoes, Vegetables, Fruit, and Nuts

You can make this salad as simple as you want and as full of extras as you wish. It all starts with lettuce.

Serves 2

INGREDIENTS

2 cups lettuce from pre-washed packaged lettuce or from washed head of lettuce, leaves torn, dark leaves preferred

10 grape or cherry tomatoes, halved

½ cup onion, sliced, optional

1 cup vegetables from pre-washed packaged vegetables such as carrots, broccoli, cabbage, mushrooms, and vegetables of your choice or from cut-up vegetables you have on hand, optional

½ cup roasted nuts, unsalted, such as walnuts, almonds, or your choice, optional

½ cup fruit such as halved grapes, optional

1 tablespoon salad dressing from bottled such as low-salt and low-fat Caesar or Italian or Homemade, recipe page 83

Salt and pepper to taste

METHOD

1. If using a head of lettuce, wash leaves and tear 2 cups. Place lettuce in a large bowl.

2. Add all other ingredients except salad dressing. Pour salad dressing over the salad, and toss.

3. Adjust amount of salad dressing to your taste. Salt and pepper to taste. Serve.

Whole Wheat Baguette

If you have baguette slices in the freezer, remove two and reheat on warm in a toaster oven for about 4 to 5 minutes, or until warmed and defrosted. Serve with extra virgin olive oil, if desired.

If you do not have any remaining cut pieces, use method for buying, slicing, and freezing baguette, recipe page 84.

Broiled Pineapple Slices
Serves 2-4

INGREDIENTS

1 can pineapple slices in juice with no added sugar

or

2-4 fresh pineapple slices, available in produce section

1 cup vanilla ice milk or vanilla frozen yogurt

METHOD

1. If using canned pineapple slices, drain opened can and reserve juice for future use.

2. Move oven rack to highest level under broiler if using oven and preheat on broil setting. Alternatively, use a toaster oven.

3. On a rimmed cookie sheet or toaster oven tray lined with aluminum foil, place 2 to 4 canned or fresh pineapple slices side by side.

4. Broil for about 3 minutes, turn with a spatula, and broil the other side until pineapple begins to brown.

5. Remove from oven and place on plates. Top with ¼ to ½ cup ice milk or frozen yogurt. Serve while warm

Light Meal

Toasted Cheese with Tomato Slice
Serves 2

INGREDIENTS

>2 teaspoons lite mayonnaise
>
>2 slices whole grain bread
>
>2 slices reduced-fat cheese such as mozzarella or Swiss
>
>2 slices from a large tomato, if available

METHOD

6. Cover toaster oven tray with aluminum foil. Spread lite mayonnaise onto each of two bread slices. Place cheese and then tomato on each slice of bread.

7. Put the cookie sheet into the oven or the tray into a toaster oven. Toast until the cheese begins to melt and the bread turns brown. Remove with a spatula onto plates.

Broccoli Slaw

Serves 2 or More

INGREDIENTS

½ package uncooked and pre-washed packaged broccoli slaw that sometimes contains other fresh items such as diced cabbage, carrots, and other vegetables

1 teaspoon Homemade Salad Dressing, recipe page 83, or bottled low-fat, low-salt salad dressing such as Italian or Caesar

1 teaspoon lite mayonnaise or plain low-fat, fat-free yogurt

METHOD

1. Place all ingredients in small bowl. Toss to mix well. Serve on small plates beside sandwiches.

2. Reserve remaining un-mixed broccoli slaw and other vegetables in the refrigerator for future use.

SNACKS

Granola Bar, High Protein

Purchase snack bars that are high in protein, low in fat, and low in sugar. Enjoy one bar per snack.

Hummus and Cut Vegetables (Crudités)

Purchase containers of prepared hummus or follow directions for Homemade Hummus, recipe page 192. If buying pre-mixed, commercial hummus, look for the least salty. Use cut-up pre-washed packaged vegetables of your choice, such as celery, carrots, cauliflower, and broccoli, to dip into the hummus. Eat about ½ cup of vegetables per snack. You can save both vegetables and hummus for future snacking.

Day 6 Menus

BREAKFAST

➢ Whole Grain English Muffins with Eggs over Light

➢ Peaches, Canned or Frozen, with Vanilla Yogurt

➢ Coffee, Tea, Milk, or Water

MAIN MEAL

➢ Sautéed Tilapia Fillets

➢ Roasted Acorn Squash, Winter Squash[1]

➢ Roasted Carrots[2]

➢ Simple Salad

➢ Whole Wheat Baguette

➢ Angel Food Cake with Peaches and Vanilla Frozen Yogurt

[1]You can use other winter squash in this recipe, such as delecta. Adjust the cooking time to the size of the halved squash.

[2]You can roast many vegetables, such as carrots, broccoli, cauliflower, yellow squash, zucchini, Brussels sprouts, and even tomatoes, eggplants, and others. When you roast these vegetables, either sprinkle them with extra virgin olive oil or canola oil or place in a bowl, add the oil, and stir the cut vegetables gently to cover in oil. Roasting vegetables, an easy way to serve and eat, brings out their natural sweetness and is a convenient way to cook vegetables when you are baking other foods.

LIGHT MEAL

➢ Sautéed White Beans with Brown Rice or Couscous

➢ Shredded Carrot Salad

SNACKS

➤ Hard Boiled Egg Segments with Tomatoes and Whole Grain Crackers

➤ Cottage Cheese and Fruit

Day 6 Recipes

BREAKFAST

Whole Grain English Muffins with Eggs over Light
Serves 2

INGREDIENTS

1 whole grain English muffin

2 teaspoons soft-tub margarine

2 teaspoons extra virgin olive oil or canola oil

2 eggs

METHOD

1. Split English muffin into two pieces and place cut-side up on tray in toaster oven. Toast and then spread with soft-tub margarine at the last minute just before egg is done. Lay ½ English muffin on each plate.

2. Break eggs into a small bowl, one at a time.

3. Heat oil in a non-stick frying pan on medium heat. When pan is heated, add and cook eggs one at a time.

4. When the white begins to firm, turn egg and cook for about 30 seconds to 1 minute longer.

5. Remove the egg from the pan and place on top of toasted English muffin half. Repeat with second egg.

Peaches, Canned or Frozen, with Vanilla Yogurt

Serves 2

INGREDIENTS

**1 cup sliced peaches from 1 can or 1 package frozen
and defrosted, containing no added sugar**

½ cup or 1 8-ounce carton vanilla yogurt

METHOD

1. Open canned or thawed frozen packaged peaches. Drain, if necessary, reserving juice for future use.

2. Add ½ cup peaches in each of 2 small bowls. Top with ¼ cup low-fat or fat-free vanilla yogurt.

3. Serve beside the English muffins, eggs, and drinks of your choice.

MAIN MEAL

Note that the preparation order of the following dishes for the Main Meal recipes insures that the dishes are ready at about the same time.

Roasted Acorn Squash, Winter Squash
Serves 2-4

INGREDIENTS

1 acorn squash, as green as possible, or any 1 winter squash

2 teaspoons extra virgin olive oil or canola oil

2 teaspoons maple syrup, honey, or brown sugar

2 teaspoons raisins

2 teaspoons roasted slivered almonds, optional

METHOD

1. Pre-heat oven to 400 degrees.

2. Pick one deep-green acorn squash for two servings. If using another variety of winter squash, adjust number selected according to size. Wash thoroughly.

3. Carefully slice the acorn squash in half, lengthwise. Clean out the seeds[1] with a spoon.

4. Place the pre-washed squash in a baking dish or pan after slicing a thin piece off the bottom to ensure that it sits level.

5. Mix oil; maple syrup, honey or brown sugar; raisins; and optional nuts in a small bowl and place half the mixture in each cleaned cavity of the squash.

6. Pour about ½ inch of water into the pan or dish with the squash in order to keep it from scorching or sticking to the pan.

7. Place the pan into the preheated oven. Roast the squash until it is fork tender, about an hour.

[1]**Seeds:** You can prepare the seeds from the squash for snacking by washing them and roasting them at the same time you bake the squash. Add a small amount of salt-free butter and a couple of shakes of salt to the pan where the seeds are evenly spread in one layer. Roast until slightly brown.

Roasted Carrots

Serves 4-6

INGREDIENTS

3 whole carrots or 10 baby carrots

1 tablespoon extra virgin olive oil or canola oil

1 teaspoon dried tarragon

2 teaspoons vinegar, Balsamic, apple cider, white, or your choice

Salt to taste

METHOD

1. Pre-heat oven to 400 degrees.

2. Scrape and wash the whole carrots. Cut into 2- to 3-inch pieces.

3. Place 1 tablespoon oil in a large bowl. Add the dried tarragon and vinegar. Put in cut carrots or the baby carrots. Swirl carrots in the oil mixture until all are covered. Sprinkle salt over the oiled carrots.

4. Place oiled and salted carrots on an aluminum-foil-lined baking sheet with rims and roast in a 400 degrees oven for about 40 to 50 minutes or until tender.

5. Remove roasted carrots from oven and serve with the rest of the Main Meal.

Recipe tested by Meredith Downing

Simple Salad

Serves 2

INGREDIENTS

    2 cups pre-washed packaged lettuce or torn leaves from a head of lettuce, dark leaves preferred

    10 grape or cherry tomatoes, halved

    2 teaspoons from low-fat, low-salt bottled salad dressing such as Caesar or Italian or from Homemade Salad Dressing, recipe page 83

    Salt and pepper to taste

METHOD

1. Place lettuce pieces in a large bowl with the tomato halves.

2. Add salad dressing, salt, and pepper. Adjust seasonings to taste. Serve.

Whole Wheat Baguette

Serves 2

INGREDIENTS

    2 slices leftover baguette from freezer

    2 teaspoons extra virgin olive oil

METHOD

1. Pre-heat oven to 350 degrees or set toaster oven to warm.

2. Spread extra virgin olive oil on the sliced baguette. Place on an aluminum-foil-lined cookie sheet or toaster oven tray. Bake, not toast, for about 5 minutes until slightly browned.

3. Remove and serve with dinner.

Sautéed Tilapia Fillets

"It was just dandy!" Kathy Cain Parkins

Serves 2

INGREDIENTS

⅓ cup whole wheat or whole grain flour and ⅓ cup cornmeal

Salt and pepper to taste

1 tablespoon extra virgin olive oil or canola oil, or as needed

½ pound tilapia or other white flesh fish such as flounder, halibut, or trout. Use either fresh or flash-frozen.

METHOD

1. Combine flour, cornmeal, salt, and pepper in a shallow dish or plate. Thoroughly dredge fillet in flour and cornmeal mixture. Discard any remaining mixture.

2. Heat oil in large, non-stick skillet over medium-high heat. When hot, add fillet and cook until lightly browned and opaque in center. Turn. Cook about 3 to 4 minutes per side.

3. Serve immediately with salad and roasted squash or carrots.

Recipe tested by Kathy Cain Parkins

Angel Food Cake with Peaches and Vanilla Frozen Yogurt

Serves 2

INGREDIENTS

2 slices angel food cake, 1-2 inches thick, from freezer or cut from whole cake

1 cup frozen or canned peaches packed in fruit juice

1 cup vanilla frozen yogurt

METHOD

Place 1 slice angel food cake on each of 2 plates. Top with ½ cup drained peaches and ½ cup vanilla frozen yogurt. Serve.

LIGHT MEAL

Sautéed White Beans with Brown Rice or Couscous

This is a colorful recipe when you use the fresh parsley, halved tomatoes, diced banana or wax peppers, and fresh oregano leaves.

Serves 2

INGREDIENTS

2 teaspoons extra virgin olive oil or canola oil

2 teaspoons onion powder or dried minced onion or ½ cup onion, chopped

1 teaspoon garlic powder or dried minced garlic or 1 clove garlic, chopped

1 teaspoon ground cumin, optional

¼ cup beef, chicken, or vegetable broth, or white wine

1 can white beans, such as navy, cannellini, or great northern white, rinsed and drained to remove excess salt, or 1 cup cooked dried beans from 16-ounce package, recipe page 225

2 teaspoons dried oregano or 1 tablespoon fresh oregano leaves

2 teaspoons dried parsley or 3 tablespoons fresh parsley, minced or chopped

½ cup grape or cherry tomatoes, halved

¼ cup banana or wax peppers, chopped, optional

Salt and pepper to taste, using a minimum of salt

METHOD

1. Add oil to a saucepan over medium heat. When the oil is hot, add the fresh onion, if using, and sauté until soft, about 5 minutes. Add the fresh garlic, if using, and cumin and cook until fragrant, about 2 minutes.

2. If using powdered or dried minced onion and garlic, add at this time with the cumin.

3. Immediately add the broth or white wine and raise the heat. Cook until the liquid has reduced by half.

4. Stir in the beans, oregano, parsley, tomatoes, and banana or wax pepper. Season with salt and pepper to taste.

5. Cook gently for 15 minutes. Transfer to a serving bowl and serve with brown rice, page 80, or couscous, page 81.

Recipe tested by Ruth Porter

Carrot Salad
Serves 2

INGREDIENTS

**Lemon juice from ½ lemon, 1 tablespoon bottled
pure lemon juice, or 1 tablespoon Balsamic,
apple cider, white, or vinegar of your choice**

½ teaspoon honey

1 tablespoon extra virgin olive oil or canola oil

Salt and pepper to taste

¼ cup raisins

**1 cup pre-washed packaged shredded or chopped
carrots, or 2 whole carrots, shredded in a food
processor or hand-held grater**

METHOD

1. In a salad bowl, mix lemon juice or vinegar, honey, oil, salt, and pepper.

2. Add raisins and carrots and toss well. Adjust seasonings to taste. Divide and serve in 2 bowls.

SNACKS

Hard Boiled Egg Segments with Tomatoes and Whole Grain Crackers
Serves 2

INGREDIENTS

1 egg, or more for more servings

1 medium tomato, 4 grape tomatoes, or 2 cherry tomatoes

1 large whole grain cracker

METHOD

1. Boil 1 or more eggs according to recipe on page 224. Refrigerated hard boiled eggs, kept in the shell, can be kept for 1 week, and they make excellent snacks.

2. Peel, rinse, and slice 1 hard boiled egg in half or quarters. Serve with tomato segments, grape, or cherry tomatoes; and whole grain cracker.

Cottage Cheese and Fruit
Serves 2

INGREDIENTS

1 cup low-fat or fat-free cottage cheese

1 cup fruit, your choice, fresh or frozen or canned packed in fruit juice

METHOD

Place ½ cup cottage cheese into each of 2 small bowls. Add ½ cup fruit of your choice, fresh, canned, or frozen.

Chapter 14

Staying Healthy

Eating at Fast Food Outlets or Restaurants

Ordering and eating out is a way of life for many, especially when you're too tired or too busy to cook. But you can make the same healthy choices that are becoming a regular part of your new healthy lifestyle. Congratulate yourself!

Here are some guidelines you can use to make sure you stick with a healthy diet.

- Try Subway's healthy sandwiches, not those that are high fat and high salt. Buy them small sized.

- Order salads or grilled chicken and fish, never fried foods.

- Order meats and fish grilled with no added butters and oils.

- Order salad dressing on the side, adding only as much as you need. You can dip your fork into the dressing to accompany each bite of undressed salad.

- Avoid mayonnaise and other full-fat salad dressings or condiments.

- Choose low-fat or reduced-fat cheese or request half the amount of cheese that is offered with the meal. Take home the rest.

185

- Patronize fast food outlets that offer healthy foods, such as Panera Bread, Au Bon Pain, Noodles and Company, Jason's Deli, and others. Avoid salty, highly sweetened, fried, fatty foods, and sodas—both sugared and diet—and sweet tea. In particular, avoid the popular French fries and unending sodas!

- Don't use the buffet because you'll tend to eat too much. Also you don't know how long the food has been sitting out there.

- Take home some of your meal. You can ask for half the meal to be boxed up even before the server brings your plate to you. This strategy helps prevent over-indulging, plus you've save some prepared food for a future meal.

Chapter 15

Celebrations!

Menus, Recipes, and Ideas

Celebrations are meant to be fun! We're with family and friends, and we're around a table with good, healthy food and good feelings. These are the days that we celebrate meaningful times—religious holidays, birthdays, anniversaries, graduations, births, and on and on.

We can have the fun of a celebration and still be true to our healthy lifestyle and healthy eating. All the while doing it in as easy a way as possible.

The Celebrations! chapter focuses on the main dish, usually a roast, because it's easy and celebratory. If you prefer, you may choose any dish from your "Healthy Eating Plan" menus.

After that main dish, there are suggested appetizers, side dishes, and desserts that will go well with the entrées or you can also select any dish from the "Healthy Eating Plan." Only your budget, the number of guests, their dietary preferences, and the season will limit your choices.

Have fun while you celebrate—and stay healthy!

Celebrations!

MENU SUGGESTIONS

SUPER EASY

APPETIZERS

➢ Shrimp, cooked, shelled, with or without tails, shrimp cocktail sauce

➢ Sticks of firm vegetables (crudités) such as celery, bell peppers, broccoli, carrots, and snow pea pods. (You can buy these already prepared in the produce section of the grocery store.)

> Dips for vegetable sticks, bread sticks, toast bits, or pita wedges
>
> Sour cream with horseradish
>
> Hummus

➢ Nuts and Seeds, roasted and seasoned

> Dusted lightly with cayenne, onion salt, or sugar

➢ Asparagus spears, roasted

➢ Olives, stuffed with pimento, or other foods

➢ Deviled Eggs

SALADS

➢ Spinach, baby leaves, with strawberries or grapes (for Winter)

➢ Bibb lettuce with onions and mushrooms (for Spring)

➢ Sliced tomatoes with goat cheese or Parmesan (for Summer)

➢ Salads with lettuce of your choice (Pre-washed packaged lettuce is an easy way to make salad.) and additions to salads, including nuts, seeds, fruits, and any number of vegetables

ENTRÉES

➤ Roasts with Gravy or Sauce
    Chicken
    Turkey
    Pork
    Lamb
    Salmon

SIDES

➤ Green beans, Brussels sprouts, fresh lima beans, green peas, roasted asparagus, or green vegetable of your choice (Canned or frozen is Super Easy.)

➤ Sautéed yellow squash, zucchini, bell pepper, or other vegetable with onions and garlic (Summer)

➤ Roasted carrots

➤ Roasted asparagus (Spring)

SUPER EASY

➤ Baked sweet potato circles or wedges

➤ Brown rice, couscous, or whole grain of your choice

➤ Cranberry sauce

DESSERTS

SUPER EASY

➤ Angel food cake topped with chocolate sauce, strawberries, bananas, or fruit of your choice; ice milk or frozen yogurt

➤ Crustless pies, including peach, berry, and pumpkin

➤ Blender Fruit Whip

BEVERAGES FOR CELEBRATIONS!

➤ White or red wine, depending on your entrée

➤ Iced tea

➤ Chilled water

➤ Coffee or Hot Tea

Celebrations!

RECIPES

APPETIZERS

Shrimp with Bottled Shrimp Cocktail Sauce
Serves 4

INGREDIENTS

1 pound medium- or small-sized shelled shrimp, deveined, and tail on or 1 ½ pound shrimp with shells

1 lemon or 1 tablespoon bottled pure lemon juice

1 bottle shrimp cocktail sauce

METHOD

1. If you are working with cooked and deveined shrimp, squeeze or pour the lemon juice over the shrimp and place in the refrigerator until ready to serve.

2. If shrimp are not cooked, boil them in their shells in water until the shells turn pink. Cool until you are able to handle the cooked shrimp. Remove the shells, but leave the tails on, if you wish. With a sharp pointed knife, open the back of the shrimp to expose the vein. Remove the vein with the point of the knife. Squeeze or pour the lemon juice over all the peeled shrimp. Place the shrimp in the refrigerator to cool until ready to serve.

3. Arrange the shelled shrimp on a plate or in a bowl and serve with the shrimp sauce in a small bowl on the side for dipping. (This sauce is high in salt and may contain high fructose sugar. Use very little for each dipped shrimp.)

Vegetable Sticks (Crudités) with Dips

Serves 4-6

INGREDIENTS

Firm vegetables that you prepare, or from pre-washed packaged vegetables of your choice such as any of the following:

Celery

Bell peppers

Broccoli

Carrots

Snow peas

METHOD

1. If using pre-washed packaged vegetables, remove a total of 1 to 2 cups from the packages and place on a plate beside the dips.

2. If preparing your own vegetables, wash each vegetable. Halve the bell peppers and remove the pith and seeds. Remove the tough part of the broccoli stem. Scrape the carrots, if necessary. Remove the stem on the snow peas. Prepare the other vegetables as needed.

3. Slice each vegetable into 2 to 3 inch sticks and arrange neatly on a serving dish beside the dips.

Bread Pieces for Dips

Serves 4-6

INGREDIENTS

Bread sticks	**Toast wedges**
Pita wedges	**Crackers**

METHOD

Buy whole grain breads, crackers, or sticks with little or no added fats, sugar, or salt. Arrange them on a serving plate or container. Place dips nearby.

DIPS

Sour Cream with Horseradish
Serves 4

INGREDIENTS

>**1 cup low-fat sour cream**
>
>**1 tablespoon horseradish**
>
>**Salt to taste**

METHOD

Place ingredients in a small bowl. Mix thoroughly. Serve beside the prepared vegetable sticks and bread pieces.

Hummus

This is ready-made or easily made in a blender or food processor.
Serves 4-6

PURCHASED

Buy 1 container hummus, your choice of flavors. Be careful to avoid high salt content.

HOMEMADE

INGREDIENTS

>**⅓ to ½ cup Tahini (sesame seed paste), available in foreign food section of the grocery store, optional**
>
>**1 16-ounce can chick peas with the liquid reserved**
>
>**⅓ cup lemon juice from fresh lemons or bottled pure lemon juice**
>
>**2 teaspoons powdered or dried minced garlic or 2 cloves garlic, peeled and chopped**
>
>**Salt to taste**

METHOD

1. Traditional, Middle Easter hummus uses Tahini, but this dish can be made without this sesame seed paste. If using the Tahini, place it and all the other ingredients in the bowl of a blender, an immersion or handheld blender, or food processor. Otherwise, omit the Tahini and proceed with other ingredients.

2. The lemon juice not only adds flavor to the hummus, it also thickens the mixture when Tahini is used. Blend until all the ingredients are thoroughly mixed and smooth.

3. Add liquid from the canned chickpeas when necessary for the mixture to blend well. Be careful that the mixture does not become too liquid.

4. You may have to use a rubber spatula to scrape down the sides of the bowl. Taste and adjust seasonings as needed.

5. Scrape the mixed hummus into a bowl and place beside the vegetable sticks and bread pieces of your choice. Reserve the remainder in a closed container for future use as a snack.

Seasoned Nuts

Serves 4-6

INGREDIENTS

2 cups roasted nuts of your choice (Buy raw nuts. Available in produce section of grocery store.)

1 teaspoon cayenne pepper

1 teaspoon onion salt

Or

1 teaspoon dark or light brown sugar

METHOD

1. Pre-heat the oven to 350 degrees. Spread the raw nuts in a single layer on a rimmed cookie sheet. Place in the oven and bake for 8 to 9 minutes. Remove and cool. (These roasted nuts can be reserved for snacks, salads, or other uses. They are very nutritious. Buying them this way is most economical.)

2. Place 1 cup of the roasted nuts in a bowl and sprinkle with the cayenne pepper and onion salt. Toss and serve.

3. Place another 1 cup of the roasted nuts in a second bowl. Sprinkle with the brown sugar. Toss and serve.

4. Reserve the leftover roasted nuts in closed containers for future use as a snack, with salads, cereals, and other dishes.

Salted Seeds
Serves 4-6

INGREDIENTS

2 cups roasted seeds of your choice (Buy raw, unsalted seeds. Available in the produce section of the grocery store.)

2 teaspoons extra virgin olive oil or canola oil

1 teaspoon unsalted butter

Salt to taste

METHOD

1. Pre-heat oven to 350 degrees.

2. In a bowl, toss 1 package of raw seeds with the oil till they are covered. Add more oil if necessary.

3. Place raw, oiled seeds in one layer on a rimmed cookie sheet or in a baking pan. Add unsalted butter to the pan.

4. Bake for 8 to 10 minutes until browned and crisp, but not burned. Remove from oven and cool.

5. Put 2 cups of the roasted seeds in a bowl and sprinkle with salt to taste. Serve.

6. Save leftovers in a closed container for snacks.

Roasted Asparagus Spears

Serves 4-6

INGREDIENTS

1 bunch fresh asparagus (One bunch will serve a number of people. Save leftovers for future use in salads or as snacks.)

2 teaspoons extra virgin olive oil or canola oil

Salt to taste

METHOD

1. Preheat the oven to 400 degrees. Wash the asparagus. Grasp the bottom of each spear in one hand and the top in the other hand. Bend the spear and the tough part will snap off.

2. In a bowl, add the oil and the top parts of the spears. Toss until they are covered in oil.

3. Place in one layer on a rimmed cookie sheet that is covered in aluminum foil and roast about 25 minutes or until beginning to brown.

4. Remove from the oven and cool. Sprinkle with salt to taste and arrange on a serving dish.

Olives with Pimento or Other Stuffings

Serves 4-6

INGREDIENTS

1 bottle stuffed green olives, or olives of your choice (These can be stuffed with almonds, garlic, anchovies, or other food items.)

METHOD

Drain vinegar from the bottle and rinse the olives. Place the rinsed and drained olives on a serving dish. Offer toothpicks beside the olive dish.

Deviled Eggs
Serves 6-8

INGREDIENTS

5-6 eggs

1 tablespoon low-fat or fat-free Greek yogurt

1 tablespoon low-fat or fat-free sour cream

1 tablespoon pickled relish, sweet or sour

Salt to taste

Sprinkles of paprika for garnish

METHOD

1. Use eggs that are a few days old. Very fresh eggs are hard to peel. Place the eggs on the bottom of a pan without crowding. Cover with 1-inch cold water above the eggs. Place on a burner and bring to a full boil.

2. When the water starts a full, rolling boil, immediately remove the pan from the burner and cover. Allow the eggs to sit in the hot water for 15 minutes. In a sink, pour the hot water from the pan and run cold water over the eggs until they feel cool.

3. To peel, gently crack the shell on a counter top, beginning to pull the peel off at the large end. Pick off the shell slowly so you don't mar the whites.

4. Place the peeled, rinsed eggs on a cutting board and halve the long way with a sharp knife. Push the yolks out of the halved eggs into a bowl.

5. Add the Greek yogurt, sour cream, relish, and salt. Mash with a fork and thoroughly mix.

6. With a spoon, place the mixture into the cavity formed when you removed the yolk. Sprinkle with the paprika and arrange on a serving dish.

SALADS

Spinach Salad with Strawberries or Grapes
Serves 4-6

INGREDIENTS

**1-2 packages of pre-washed baby spinach leaves or
1 bunch baby spinach**

**½ cup sliced purple onion or chopped onion of your
choice**

**1 cup fresh strawberries or seedless grapes, your
choice**

**1 tablespoon salad dressing, either bottled low-salt,
low-fat, such as Caesar or Italian or Homemade
Salad Dressing, recipe page 83**

Salt and pepper to taste

METHOD

1. Wash spinach leaves if not pre-washed and dry with a paper towel. Tear the leaves into bite-size pieces. Place in a bowl large enough for the spinach and other items.

2. Peel the purple onion or onion of your choice. Slice and place in the bowl with the spinach.

3. Wash the strawberries or grapes thoroughly. Remove green stems and leaves. Cut into 2 or 3 pieces. Place them in the bowl with the spinach.

4. Add the salad dressing and adjust the amount to your taste. Add salt and pepper to taste. Toss and serve as the first course or with the dinner.

Bibb Lettuce Salad with Onions and Mushrooms

Bibb lettuce is a fragile lettuce and goes well with spring celebratory meals.

Serves 4-6

INGREDIENTS

1-2 heads of Bibb lettuce, often available in a plastic, protective container in the produce section

½ cup sliced white onions or onions of your choice

1 cup white mushrooms, available pre-sliced

1 small tomato, vine ripe if possible

1 tablespoon salad dressing, either bottled low-salt, low-fat Caesar or Italian or Homemade Salad Dressing, recipe page 83

METHOD

1. Remove the Bibb lettuce leaves from the head and wash, drain, and gently dry with paper towels.

2. Place the torn lettuce leaves in a bowl large enough to contain all the ingredients. Add mushrooms and onions.

3. Add salad dressing and adjust the amount to your taste. Toss gently so you don't bruise the lettuce leaves. Serve.

Sliced Tomato Salad with Goat Cheese or Parmesan

Serves 4-6

INGREDIENTS

2-3 tomatoes, depending on size, vine ripe if possible

Salt and pepper to taste

1 cup crumbled goat cheese or shredded Parmesan cheese

1 tablespoon salad dressing, adjusting the amount to your taste

METHOD

1. Wash and slice across the wide part of the tomatoes. Lay the slices on a platter or plate for each guest.

2. Pour the salad dressing over the tomatoes. Sprinkle the tomatoes with goat cheese crumbles or shredded Parmesan cheese and salt, as needed. Serve on a platter or plates for each person.

ENTRÉES

When you buy meats to be roasted, they may seem expensive. So always buy when there is a sale, and place the roast in the freezer until ready to use. Also, there will be leftovers that you can use for soups, stews, sandwiches, and snacks.

You can use any of the Main Meal entrees in the "Menus! Recipes!," and in "More Healthy, Easy Recipes" instead of the following recipes.

Roast Whole Chicken
Serves 4-6

INGREDIENTS

> 1 roasting chicken, 5-6 pounds or as needed
>
> Juice of 1 lemon, 1 tablespoon bottled pure lemon juice or 1 tablespoon vinegar such as white, apple cider, or Balsamic
>
> 1-2 teaspoons dried herbs or 1 tablespoon fresh herbs, such as tarragon and basil
>
> 1 teaspoon powdered garlic or minced dried garlic or 1 clove garlic peeled and chopped
>
> Lemon pepper to taste
>
> 1-2 teaspoons paprika
>
> Salt to taste, keeping it to a minimum
>
> 1 onion, peeled and cut into quarters
>
> 10 baby carrots or 1 whole carrot, scraped and cut into 2- to 3-inch pieces
>
> 1 cup low-salt, reduced-fat chicken broth, 1 cup white wine, or 1 cup other liquid such as apple juice

METHOD

1. Preheat the oven to 450 degrees. Remove any packet of giblets inside the chicken. Sauté the liver to serve with the chicken and freeze the rest to use for making stock or soup.

2. Rinse the chicken inside and out. Pat dry with a paper towel. Halve the lemon and squeeze the juice into the chicken's cavity or add the bottled lemon juice or vinegar. Place the lemon halves, if any, inside the cavity. Add the fresh or dried herbs and the garlic to the cavity.

3. Place chicken, breast-side up, in an oiled roasting pan. Before placing in the oven, sprinkle the chicken with more dried herbs, lemon pepper, paprika, and salt to taste, keeping the salt to a minimum.

4. Peel and quarter the onion, placing the quarters in the pan next to the chicken. Add the baby carrots or scrape and wash the whole carrot and cut into 1- to 2-inch pieces. Place the carrots beside the chicken.

5. Roast for 1 hour and remove the chicken from the oven. Let rest on a plate or cutting board for 10 minutes before cutting or slicing.

6. To make a sauce, spoon out most of the fat from the roasting pan and then place the pan on a burner on top of the stove. Add 1 cup chicken broth or other liquid to the pan. Bring to a boil, scraping the bottom of the pan with a wooden spoon. Reduce the liquid by half by boiling.

7. Serve in a bowl with the meal to pour over the chicken pieces or brown rice, if using.

MENU SUGGESTIONS FOR ROAST WHOLE CHICKEN:

Appetizers: Vegetable sticks (crudités) and sour cream dip, olives, and deviled eggs

Salads: Sliced tomatoes with goat cheese or Parmesan, Bibb lettuce salad with onions and mushrooms

Sides: Brown rice, steamed green beans, roasted sweet potato wedges

Desserts: Crustless Fruit Pie, Vanilla Ice Milk with Strawberries

Roast Turkey Breast

Turkey breast has less saturated fat than the whole chicken or turkey, and when roasted carefully can be moist and delicious.

Serves 4-6

INGREDIENTS

> **1 8-pound or less turkey breast, with or without bones. Make sure there is enough to have leftovers. (These leftovers are delicious.)**
>
> **2 tablespoons extra virgin olive oil or canola oil**
>
> **2 teaspoons dried or 1 tablespoon fresh chopped herbs such as basil, oregano, rosemary, thyme, or sage**
>
> **2 teaspoons garlic powder, dried minced garlic, or 2 cloves garlic, peeled and chopped**
>
> **2 teaspoons paprika**
>
> **Salt and pepper to taste**

METHOD

1. Preheat oven to 425 degrees. Mix the oil and herbs, either dried or fresh, pepper, garlic, paprika, salt, and pepper in a small bowl.

2. Place the turkey breast in a roasting pan. With your hands, thoroughly spread the oil and herbs mixture all over the turkey breast.

3. Place the turkey breast in the pre-heated oven so the skin-side is up in the oiled roasting pan. Roast for about 45 to 55 minutes until an instant read thermometer reads 165 degrees or the juices run clear when pricked with a fork in the thickest part. If there are bones in your turkey breast, be sure the thermometer does not touch a bone.

4. Remove from the oven, cover loosely with aluminum foil, and let rest for about 10 minutes before slicing or carving.

5. Place sliced turkey breast on a platter and serve with vegetables and cranberry sauce (page 213-214).

MENU SUGGESTIONS FOR ROAST TURKEY BREAST
As a Thanksgiving or Christmas dish, turkey goes well with:

Appetizers: Nuts and seeds, roasted and seasoned; bread pieces with hummus dip; stuffed olives

Salads: Spinach salad with strawberries or grapes, lettuce with vegetables, fruit, and nuts

Sides: Sweet potato wedges, roasted Brussels sprouts, homemade cranberry sauce

Desserts: Pumpkin pudding, strawberry ice milk or frozen yogurt with angel food cake

Roast Pork Loin

This is a simple recipe for a lean cut of pork, usually served in the fall or winter, though it works well any time of the year.

Serves 4-6

INGREDIENTS

1 3-pound pork loin, trimmed of fat and secured with string (The grocery store has pork loin already trimmed and tied with string. If possible avoid pre-seasoned pork as it is often high salt.)

Salt and pepper to taste

4 teaspoons powdered garlic or minced dried garlic or 3 cloves garlic, peeled and chopped

2 tablespoons extra virgin olive oil or canola oil

2 teaspoons dried rosemary or 2 tablespoons chopped fresh rosemary

1 tablespoon freshly grated lemon zest, optional

¾ cup vegetable broth, apple juice, or white wine

2 tablespoons vinegar, such as apple cider, white, or Balsamic

METHOD

1. If you have pork loin that is not already prepared by the grocery store, trim the fat and tie kitchen string around pork loin in three places to prevent it from flattening while roasting.

2. Place about 1 teaspoon salt and garlic in a small bowl.

3. If using lemon zest, slide a whole lemon over the small grates of a grater to remove the zest, which is the yellow portion of the peel, not the white. Add the zest to the garlic and salt mixture. Add the oil and fresh or dried rosemary. Mix well and with your hands rub the mixture all over the pork loin. Refrigerate for 1 hour.

4. Preheat oven to 375 degrees. Remove the pork loin from the refrigerator and place in an oiled roasting pan. Roast for about 40 to 50 minutes, uncovered and turning once or twice, until a thermometer inserted into the thickest part registers 145 degrees or until the inner flesh has a very slight pink hue. Transfer to a cutting board and let rest for 10 minutes before slicing or carving.

5. Meanwhile, spoon off and discard most of the melted fat from the roasting pan and add broth, apple juice, or wine to the pan. Place the pan over medium-high heat on top of the stove and bring to a simmer, scraping up any browned bits. Simmer until the sauce is reduced by half, about 2 to 4 minutes.

6. After the pork loin has rested on the cutting board for 10 minutes, remove the string and slice the roast into serving-size pieces. Place the sliced pieces on a platter and serve.

7. Pour juices from the cutting board into the sauce and pour the finished sauce into a bowl. Place the sauce on the table to serve over the pork and/or accompanying sides.

MENU SUGGESTIONS FOR ROAST PORK LOIN

Appetizers: Vegetable sticks (crudités) with sour cream dip, stuffed olives, or seasoned nuts

Salads: Spinach salad with strawberries or grapes; lettuce with vegetables, fruit, and nuts

Sides: Sautéed apple slices, roasted carrots, brown rice, sautéed bell
peppers with onions and garlic, and braised green beans
Desserts: Crustless fruit pie and Fruit Whip

Roast Leg of Lamb

Traditionally a spring dish, buy lamb when it is on sale and store
in the freezer or roast and serve right away. Below is a simple recipe
that I got from an Italian-Swiss family.

Serves 4-6

INGREDIENTS

**1 leg of lamb, about 8-9 pounds with bone in or 5-6
pounds boneless**

3 cloves garlic, peeled and cut into slivers

2 tablespoons whole-grain mustard

1 tablespoon dried rosemary

**10-15 baby carrots or 3 whole carrots, washed,
scraped, and cut into 1- to 3-inch pieces**

METHOD

1. Preheat oven to 350 degrees. Wash and pat dry the defrosted leg
   of lamb. Make slits all over the leg of lamb and push the slivers
   of garlic into the slits.

2. Mix the mustard with the rosemary and with your hands spread
   the mixture evenly all over the leg of lamb.

3. Place the carrots next to the lamb in an oiled baking pan and
   bake about 1 hour and 20 minutes until the instant read thermometer reads 140 degrees or the flesh is pale pink.

4. Put the roasted lamb on platter on a cutting board and let rest
   10 minutes. Meanwhile transfer the roasted carrots to the serving platter.

5. After 10 minutes, slice or carve the leg of lamb and place the
   serving-size pieces on a platter with the carrots. Reserve leftover
   lamb for future meals.

MENU SUGGESTIONS FOR ROAST LEG OF LAMB

Appetizers: Roasted asparagus spears, vegetable sticks (crudités) with sour cream dip, deviled eggs

Salads: Bibb lettuce salad with onions and mushrooms; sliced tomatoes with goat cheese or Parmesan; lettuce salad with vegetables, fruit, and nuts

Sides: Sautéed yellow squash and zucchini with onions and garlic, couscous with green peas, or other in-season vegetable

Desserts: Fruit Whip, ice milk with strawberries, cookies, and berries

Baked Salmon Fillet with Pecans

Salmon is a dish often served in the summer, but it can be served any time of year. Baked salmon is one of the simpler dishes to make. This recipe has a sauce that adds to the celebrations. You can bake several kinds for fish fillets such as cod, haddock, grouper, trout, or other oily fish.

Serves 4-6

INGREDIENTS

½ cup pecans, chopped. Pecans taste very good with salmon, but you may use other kinds of nuts.

½ cup dark brown sugar or 2 tablespoons maple syrup

2 teaspoons extra virgin olive oil or canola oil

½ cup water, vegetarian broth, or bourbon

Salt and pepper to taste

1 pound salmon fillet, cut from the thick part of the fillet, for 4-6 pieces

METHOD

1. Preheat oven to 425 degrees and cover a rimmed baking sheet with aluminum foil.

2. Place the chopped pecans in a non-stick pan over medium heat and lightly brown. Watch carefully to prevent burning.

3. Add brown sugar, 1 teaspoon oil, and water, broth, or bourbon. When the mixture begins to simmer, remove from the heat.

4. Place the salmon fillet, skin side down, on an aluminum-foil-lined, rimmed cookie sheet. Spoon half the pecan mixture over the fillet, reserving the leftover sauce for later. Put the cookie sheet with the fillet in the preheated oven and bake for 5 to 7 minutes.

5. After 5 to 7 minutes, spoon another tablespoon of the pecan mixture over the fillet and continue roasting for about 3 to 5 minutes longer, or until the salmon flakes easily with a fork.

6. Remove from the oven, turn the fillet over, and scrape the skin off with a spatula or edge of a spoon. Place the fillet on a serving plate and spoon more pecan mixture over it.

7. Serve the remaining mixture, if there is any, in a bowl to serve over the salmon or accompaniments. Reserve leftover salmon for future meals to use as sandwiches, salads, or reheated main dishes.

MENU SUGGESTIONS FOR BAKED SALMON FILLET

Appetizers: Roasted asparagus spears, vegetable sticks (crudités) with sour cream dip, seasoned nuts

Salads: Bibb lettuce salad with onions and mushrooms; sliced tomatoes with goat cheese or Parmesan; lettuce salad with vegetables, fruit, and nuts

Sides: Brown rice, fresh lima beans, green peas

Desserts: Angel food cake with strawberries, Fruit Whip

SIDES

Brown Rice

You may use pre-cooked packaged or frozen brown rice. Be sure there is little added salt and no sugar and follow package directions.

To make your own homemade brown rice, follow this simple, foolproof method that can be used for most rice recipes. Homemade brown rice is cheaper than prepared rice or boxed rice. It costs about 18 cents a serving. This recipe also appears on page 80.

Serves 4

INGREDIENTS

1 cup long-grain brown rice

1 ½ cups water or reduced-fat and low-salt beef, chicken, or vegetable broth, or mixture of water and broth

Salt and pepper, to taste, with salt kept to a minimum

METHOD

1. Add brown rice to medium-sized saucepan with the water, broth, or mixture of the two.

2. Bring to a rolling boil. Immediately turn down heat to a low simmer and cover saucepan. Check two or three times in the first minutes to make sure the water does not boil over.

3. Set timer to 45 to 50 minutes and lift lid only when the time is up. At that time, check whether the rice has absorbed all the water and that the rice is fluffy.

4. If all the water is not yet absorbed, cover and continue cooking over low heat. Check every 10 minutes until the rice is done and the water is absorbed. If the rice is uncooked and too dry, add about 2 tablespoons water and continue cooking for 10 to 15 minutes or until tender.

5. Leftover brown rice can be stored in resealable plastic bags or a covered container in the refrigerator or frozen for future use. It can be reheated in the microwave in a loosely covered bowl or plate for 1 to 2 minutes.

Couscous

Couscous is small pasta from North Africa. You can buy instant whole wheat couscous. It goes well with many main dishes and is very easy to make. For making couscous, follow the package directions or those below. This recipe is also found on page 81.

Serves 4-6

Ingredients

　　　1 teaspoon extra virgin olive oil or canola oil

　　　½ cup instant packaged whole wheat couscous

　　　¾ cup boiling water or broth or a mix of the two

　　　Salt and pepper, to taste, salt kept to a minimum

METHOD

1. Bring water or broth or the mixture to a boil in a medium saucepan. Add couscous.

2. Immediately cover and remove from heat. Allow to sit undisturbed for 5 to 10 minutes.

3. After 5 to 10 minutes, fluff the couscous gently with a fork. Serve.

4. Refrigerate or freeze leftover couscous in serving-size resealable plastic bags or plastic container to use with other dishes. Reheat by placing the couscous on a dish or in a bowl, loosely covered with a paper towel or wax paper, and heat in the microwave to 1 to1½ minutes.

Steamed Green Beans

Most vegetables can be steamed. This process tenderizes the vegetables and brings out their natural sweetness. This is a fast way to cook vegetables after they are prepared, so time them to finish cooking when the rest of the meal is ready to serve. And watch them carefully to prevent them from overcooking.

Serves 4-6

INGREDIENTS

> **1 box frozen green beans or 2 cans green beans with little or no added salt or fat, or 1 pound fresh green beans**
>
> **1 teaspoon soft-tub margarine**
>
> **Salt and pepper to taste, adding a minimum salt**

METHOD

1. If using frozen green beans, follow package directions. If using canned green beans, drain, pour out into a colander, and rinse to eliminate excess salt. Heat in a small saucepan.

2. If using fresh green beans, wash them in a colander. Cut off stem ends. Cut into about 2-inch pieces. Place enough water in a medium-size saucepan to come to the bottom of a steamer basket. Or place a minimum amount of water in the bottom of a medium saucepan.

3. Place the prepared green beans in the steamer basket or in the saucepan. Bring the water to a boil and cover. Steam for about 3 to 5 minutes, checking the beans for tenderness, but not mushy, during and after that time.

4. When the green beans are ready, place them in a bowl. Add ½ teaspoon soft-tub margarine, salt, and pepper to taste. Toss and serve.

Roasted Sweet Potato Wedges

"We used fresh rosemary and it was good. We ate them all up!!"
Angela Ebert

Sweet potatoes are high in Vitamin A, complex carbohydrates, and fiber; and are low-sodium and low-calorie. The skin is edible. This recipe is simple, adaptable, and healthy.

Serves 4-6

INGREDIENTS

2-4 small or medium-sized sweet potatoes

1 tablespoon extra virgin olive oil or canola oil

½ teaspoon each of some of the following spices and herbs:

For sweet version—ground cinnamon, ground ginger, allspice, pumpkin pie spice. You can also add 1 tablespoon brown sugar, honey, or maple syrup.

For savory—red pepper, rosemary, or sage; fresh or dried.

METHOD

1. Preheat oven to 400 degrees. Scrub the sweet potatoes clean. Dry with paper towels. On a cutting board, cut the sweet potatoes in half. Cut the halves into two to four sections, making wedges. Peel, if desired, though peeling is not necessary.

2. Place the oil and the chosen herbs or spices in a bowl or in a resealable plastic bag. Add the sweet potato wedges and swirl them around in the oil mixture with the herbs or spices until they are covered.

3. Put the wedges in one layer on an aluminum-foil-lined rimmed cookie sheet, and sprinkle with brown sugar or drip honey or maple syrup over the wedges, for the sweet version. Omit adding the sugar or honey for the savory version.

4. Place in the heated oven. Bake for about 30 minutes or more until crispy on the outside and soft inside. Cooking times may vary according to your preference for crispness or softness.

5. Serve with a roast of your choice, saving remaining wedges for future use. These are good as snacks or with future meals.

Recipe tested by Angela Eberts

Roasted Brussels Sprouts

You can roast these at the same time you're roasting the meat or fish that you've chosen for your Celebration! meal. This is a low-calorie, easy recipe.

Serves 4-6-214

INGREDIENTS

1 box frozen Brussels sprouts or 1-2 pounds fresh Brussels sprouts

1 tablespoon extra virgin olive oil or canola oil

Salt and pepper to taste

METHOD

1. Roast in the oven as you are roasting your meat. Or preheat oven to 400 degrees.

2. If using fresh, wash the Brussels sprouts and dry with a paper towel. Cut off the brown ends (stem ends) and pull off the yellow leaves.

3. Place oil in a bowl and add the fresh or frozen Brussels sprouts. Swirl around in the oil until they are covered. Put the oiled Brussels sprouts on an aluminum-foiled-lined rimmed cookie sheet and place in the oven.

4. Roast for about 35 to 40 minutes until slightly browned and crisp on the outside and tender on the inside. You can test by inserting a sharp knife or fork into the middle of a Brussels sprout.

5. Remove from the oven and place in a serving bowl, adding salt and pepper to taste.

212

Cranberry Sauce

"They both turned out very yummy!" Nicole Hayward

You can make a cooked candied version or a raw blender version. Both are excellent with turkey or chicken or with many kinds of meats. They are also good as a flavoring for plain yogurt or on sandwiches.

Version I: Cooked, Candied Cranberry Sauce

Serves 6-8

INGREDIENTS

1 12-ounce package of fresh or frozen cranberries

1 whole cinnamon stick or 1 teaspoon ground cinnamon

2 tablespoons frozen orange juice, not reconstituted, or orange juice from one orange

¾ cup packed brown sugar or more to taste

METHOD

1. Place cranberries in a medium-sizes saucepan with the cinnamon stick, orange juice and brown sugar. Bring to a boil, stirring constantly.

2. After 4 to 5 minutes the berries will begin to pop and the sauce begin to thicken. Continue to cook for another 2 to 3 minutes and then remove from heat. Cool.

3. Take out the cinnamon stick, if using, and pour the cooling sauce into a jar or plastic container. When the sauce has cooled so you can lift the jar or container, put on the lid and place into the refrigerator.

Version II: No-Cook Cranberry Orange Sauce

"I was very impressed with this recipe." Nicole Hayward

Make this version at least one day ahead of your planned use so the flavors blend and mellow. This version can be used on many kinds of meats and in plain yogurt.

Serves 6-8

INGREDIENTS

1 12-ounce package fresh or frozen cranberries

1 navel orange or 1 seeded juice orange

1 container frozen orange juice, un-reconstituted

2 tablespoons honey

METHOD

1. Wash cranberries and place in the bowl of a blender or food processor. Wash orange and cut into 4 to 6 pieces.

2. If using a navel orange, add the pieces with peel to the blender bowl, food processor, or a bowl for using the immersion or handheld blender.

3. If using a juice orange, cut open, remove the seeds and, cut away the white pith between orange segments. Do not peel. Place the orange segments with the cranberries in the bowl of the blender, food processor, or the bowl for using the immersion or handheld blender.

4. Blend or process until the cranberries and orange segments are chopped and blended. There should be no large pieces in the blender or bowl.

5. Add the honey and frozen orange juice a tablespoon at a time. Taste for desired sweetness and add more as needed. Blend after each addition, using a rubber spatula to scrape down the sides.

6. When the flavor is to your taste, scrape the mixture into a covered plastic container or a jar with a lid. Refrigerate overnight or until used.

Recipe tested by Nicole Hayward

Roasted Carrots

"This carrot recipe was very simple to make and very good."
Meredith Downing

This method can be used with many vegetables. Roasting brings out the natural sweetness of vegetables. You can also roast, following these directions, pumpkin pieces, quartered potatoes, quartered or halved onions, or other firm vegetables.

Serves 4-6

INGREDIENTS

2 16-ounce or 1 32-ounce package of "baby" carrots or 3 whole carrots

1 tablespoon extra virgin olive oil or canola oil

Salt and pepper to taste, using a minimum of salt

METHOD

1. Preheat the oven to 400 degrees.

2. If using "baby" carrots, wash and dry 1 to 2 packages of carrots, reserving extras for salads, soups, or other dishes.

3. If using whole carrots, cut off ends, wash, and scrub carrots. Using a vegetable peeler or a paring knife, scrape off the carrots' outer layer. (Some people say that thoroughly washing and scrubbing a carrot is enough so additional scraping is not necessary.) On a cutting board, cut the carrots into 2- to 3-inch pieces.

4. Put the oil and carrots in a bowl and swirl around until the carrots are completely covered in oil.

5. Place the oiled carrot pieces on an aluminum-foil-lined rimmed cookie sheet and put into the heated oven. You can also place the carrots beside a roast that you are cooking. Roast the carrots for about 30 minutes, turning once or twice.

6. The carrots are done when the outsides are browning and the insides are beginning to soften when you pierce the carrot with a sharp knife or fork. Salt and pepper to taste.

7. Place beside the roasted meat or on a serving plate.

Recipes tested by Meredith Ann Downing

Sautéed Zucchini, Onions, and Garlic

"These don't take long to cook at all." Nicole Hayward

Italians like to cook this quick and delicious dish when zucchini is in season. It's really very simple and quick and goes with many main dishes and whole grains.

Serves 2

INGREDIENTS

1 tablespoon extra virgin olive oil or canola oil

2 teaspoons powdered or 1 tablespoon dried minced onion or 1 cup fresh onion, chopped

2 teaspoons powdered garlic or dried minced garlic or 2 cloves garlic, peeled and chopped

2-4 small zucchini, fresh, washed and sliced into ¼- to ½- inch rounds, ends removed

Salt and pepper to taste, using a minimum of salt

METHOD

1. In a large non-stick skillet, add the oil to the skillet and heat on medium.

2. If using fresh onion and garlic, first add the chopped onion and sauté for about a minute. Add the chopped garlic and sauté for another minute.

3. Add the sliced zucchini. At this time, add the powdered or dried minced onion and garlic.

4. Toss all the ingredients in the skillet, cooking until the zucchini turns translucent and edges are just beginning to turn brown, about 4 or 5 minutes. Add dried onion and garlic at this time

5. Taste and adjust seasonings. Salt and pepper to your preference. Mix well. Serve with the main meal.

Recipe tested by Nicole Hayward

Sautéed Bell Peppers or Other Vegetables with Onions and Garlic

Sautéing the bell pepper or other vegetables with the onion and garlic will take about 15 minutes. The sautéing does not take much of your attention. The result is outstanding. This method of cooking vegetables is useful for many kinds of vegetables: potatoes, celery, mushrooms, broccoli, zucchini, summer squash, and green beans. Sautéed vegetables can be used with sandwiches, salads, rice, pasta, or in other dishes, and can be served as side dishes.

Serves 4-6

INGREDIENTS

1 tablespoon extra virgin olive oil or canola oil

2 bell peppers

1 cup onion, chopped

2 cloves garlic, peeled and chopped

Salt and pepper to taste

METHOD

1. Place large non-stick or cast iron skillet on medium heat. Add oil to the pan and spread the oil with a spatula.

2. Cut bell peppers in half, then quarter. With a paring knife, remove the pith and seeds. Wash out remaining seeds. Cut the bell pepper into strips. Set aside.

3. Put the chopped onion into the heated pan. Cook until translucent. Add the chopped garlic. Sautee for 1 to 2 minutes. Add bell pepper slivers. Toss.

4. Let the vegetables cook on medium heat for about 5 minutes, stirring occasionally until the bell pepper softens. Salt and pepper to taste, using a minimum amount of salt.

5. Remove from heat and serve with a roast or a dish of your choice and a whole grain.

Braised Green Beans

"Green beans and fresh basil—just a gorgeous combination to-gether. Then added red pepper flakes for serving—just superb."
Nicole Hayward

When you braise, you're adding a little moisture to a large skillet. This is a delicious and simple way to cook many kinds of vegetables, such as carrots, leeks, potatoes, broccoli, parsnips, turnips, or other firm vegetables. Be sure they are cut into small enough pieces so that the entire vegetable is cooked to your desired doneness.

Serves 4-6

INGREDIENTS

1 tablespoon extra virgin olive oil or canola oil

1 package frozen whole green beans or 1 pound fresh green beans

2 teaspoons powdered or dried minced garlic or 2 cloves garlic, peeled and chopped

⅓ cup water, broth, or white wine

1 teaspoon dried herbs of your choice, such as basil, thyme, or sage, or 1 tablespoon chopped fresh herbs

Salt and pepper, to taste, keeping salt to a minimum

METHOD

1. If using frozen whole green beans, defrost and drain. Set aside

2. If using fresh green beans, wash and cut the stem ends off. Set aside.

3. Heat a large non-stick or cast iron skillet with a lid over medium heat. Add oil to the skillet and with a spatula spread over the surface.

4. If using fresh garlic, peel and chop, adding garlic to the heated oil. Cook about 1 to 2 minutes until the garlic just softens but does not turn brown.

5. Add fresh or frozen green beans to the garlic in the skillet. Toss with a spatula. Add the water or liquid of your choice and bring to a boil. Sprinkle with the herbs of your choice.

6. Cover and lower heat to low or medium low. Allow the green beans to braise in the covered pan for about 7 to 10 minutes or until tender and most of the water or other liquid has boiled away.

7. Remove from the heat, place the green beans, or any other braised vegetable, in a serving bowl, and serve with dinner.

Recipe tested by Nicole Hayward

Lima Beans with Corn (Succotash)

You can buy lima beans already shelled in the produce section of the grocery store, frozen, or canned. With frozen or canned, be sure there is little or no added salt or sugar.

Serves 4-6

INGREDIENTS

2-3 cups shelled lima beans, 2 packages frozen with no added sugar or fats, or 2 cans lima beans

Water to cover beans in a saucepan, if using fresh

Salt and pepper to taste, using a minimum of salt

2 cups frozen, canned, or fresh corn kernels

METHOD

1. If using fresh lima beans, place shelled beans in a saucepan and cover with water. Bring to a boil, and then lower heat to a simmer. Cook for 10 to 15 minutes until the lima beans are soft and somewhat mushy. Drain the liquid and save. This is "pot liquor" and is tasty. You can use this for dipping cornbread, drinking, or using in soups or in cooking other foods.

2. If using frozen lima beans, follow package directions. If using canned, drain and rinse to eliminate as much salt as possible. Warm the canned beans in a saucepan on top of the stove or in a microwave. Set aside and keep warm.

3. To cook the corn kernels, use the same saucepan as used to cook or heat the lima beans. If using frozen, defrost and drain. If using canned, rise and drain to remove excess salt.

219

4. To use fresh corn kernels, hold a shucked ear of corn on the end in a bowl so it is vertical. Being careful not to cut your fingers, slice the corn ear downward with a knife so the kernels fall into the bowl. To get 2 cups of fresh kernels, you may have to slice off the kernels from 2 or 3 ears.

5. Place the fresh or frozen corn kernels in the saucepan and barely cover with water. Cook until tender, about 5 minutes. (Or follow package directions if using frozen corn kernels.) If using canned, warm in the saucepan.

6. Combine the cooked lima beans and corn kernels to make the Succotash dish. Salt and pepper to taste.

Green Peas

Infrequently, there are fresh green peas available in the produce section of the grocery store or at a farmers market. You can readily buy frozen or canned green peas.

Serves 4-6

INGREDIENTS

1-2 packages frozen green peas, 2-3 cans green peas, or 2 cups fresh, hulled green peas. The amount depends on the number of guests at table.

Water, broth, or white wine, as needed

1 teaspoon dried mint or 1 tablespoon fresh mint, chopped

Salt and pepper to taste

METHOD

1. If using frozen green peas, follow package directions. Or place frozen or fresh green peas in a small- to medium-sized saucepan and add just enough liquid, about ½ cup, so the green peas will not burn.

2. Bring the liquid to a boil. With a spoon gradually break up the frozen green peas, if using. Turn down the heat and simmer until done, about 4 minutes. Do not overcook. Add salt and pepper if necessary, keeping the salt to a minimum.

3. If using canned, drain the green peas, rinse to remove the excess salt, and place in a saucepan with about 1 tablespoon water or other liquid. Heat until just warm.

4. Add the mint to the green peas and stir. Taste and adjust seasonings. Serve the green peas in a bowl.

Desserts

Angel Food Cake with Strawberries

This is an easy and spectacular dessert.

Serves 4-6

Ingredients

4-6 pieces of angel food cake, about 1-2 inches thick (Adjust the number of pieces to the number of guests at table.)

1-2 pints fresh strawberries or 1-2 packages frozen strawberries with no added sugar

2 teaspoons sugar

4-6 tablespoons low-fat or fat-free Cool Whip or similar product

Method

1. Cut the number of cake pieces you'll need for dessert. Place each piece in a small bowl.

2. If using fresh strawberries, wash thoroughly, remove the stem, and cut in half or quarters, depending on their size. Place in a medium-sized bowl and sprinkle with sugar. If using frozen strawberries, defrost in time for serving dessert.

3. Put fresh or frozen strawberries on top of the angel food cake in the bowls. Place 1 tablespoon low-fat or fat-free Cool Whip or similar product on top of the strawberries and angel food cake in each bowl. Serve.

Fruit Whip

"This dish was delicious, light and elegant enough to serve to dinner guests." Angela Eberts

This low-calorie, low-fat dessert takes only minutes to prepare and seems more fancy than it is. It is served when the blended ingredients are set by cooling in the refrigerator. It is adapted from the cookbook, Joy of Cooking.

Serves 4-6

INGREDIENTS

2 cups fresh or 1-2 packages frozen fruit of, your choice. Fruits can be peaches, strawberries, blueberries, blackberries, raspberries, and so forth.

2 teaspoons sugar or honey, or to taste

2 packages gelatin, either flavorless or a favorite flavor such as lemon, peach, strawberry, and so forth. Try to match the flavor of the fruit you've chosen.

Lemon juice squeezed from 1 lemon or 1 tablespoon bottled pure lemon juice

½ cup boiling water, measured when poured into the bowl of a blender

2 cups Cool Whip, slightly thawed

METHOD

1. Place the frozen or fresh fruit in the bowl of a blender or a bowl used by an immersion or handheld blender with the sugar or honey. The amount of the fruit you use depends on the number of guests you have at table. Count on ½ cup of the finished and set Fruit Whip per person.

2. Add to the blender bowl, the gelatin, lemon juice, and boiling water. Cover and blend for about 30 to 40 seconds until the fruit is fully blended. (Be careful when blending hot or boiling water. Hold down the top firmly so it doesn't spew from the blender bowl.)

3. Pour the blended mixture into a wet dish or mold and chill in the refrigerator for at least 4 hours. Serve about ½ cup for each guest in small bowls. Reserve the remainder in the refrigerator and serve with future meals or for snacks.

Recipe tested by Angela Eberts

Chapter 16

More Healthy, Easy Recipes

BASICS

Roasted Nuts

Buy a bag of raw, unsalted nuts, your preference. Preheat oven to 350 degrees. Spread a medium or large size bag of raw nuts on a rimmed cookie sheet and place in the pre-heated oven. Set timer for 9 minutes, being careful not to leave nuts in the heat too long as they will burn. After 8 or 9 minutes, remove from the oven and cool. Remove the amount you need for a recipe and place the rest in a covered plastic container or glass jar. These will keep for months and the supply will last for a long time. Two 1-ounce servings a day will add to your nutrient load and not add to your calorie count.

Hard Boiled Eggs

Place eggs in 1 layer on the bottom of a saucepan so they aren't crowded. Cover completely with cold tap water by about 1 inch. Bring to a rolling boil over high heat. Once the water is brought to a rolling boil, reduce heat to a medium low boil and cook covered for an additional 10 minutes for a "hard boiled" egg. (For a "soft boiled" eggs, cook for 3 to 4 minutes according to preference.)

After 10 minutes, remove from heat and immediately place eggs under very cold water or in a bowl of ice water to chill promptly. This helps yolks stay bright yellow instead of turning green. Chill for a few minutes in the cold water until the egg is cooled.

To peel: crack hard boiled egg on all sides on counter, roll egg between hands to loosen shell, and remove shell by peeling away. Refrigeration is necessary for hard boiled eggs if the eggs are not to be consumed within a few hours.

Cooking Small Amounts of Pasta: A Trick

A quick method for cooking small amounts of dry pasta for 1 to 2 servings is to place about a couple of ounces of uncooked pasta in a large frying pan. Cover the dry pasta with water. Bring to a boil and cook for the amount of time called for on the package. Test for doneness about 2 minutes before the time is up. When the pasta is done, *al dente,* remove from the frying pan with tongs or a slotted spoon and place in a serving bowl, ready to serve.

Dried Beans

Buy one 16-ounce package beans of your choice. Pour the contents in a colander and rinse under running water till the water runs clear. Pick our any foreign material or stones. Place the rinsed beans in a large pot and cover with water about an inch. Let sit overnight or bring to a rapid boil and let sit for about 3 hours. After the beans have soaked, pour off the water, rinse again, and cover with about 1 inch water, broth, or a mix of the two. Bring to a boil, turn down the heat so the beans are simmering, and cook for about 2 hours until the beans are soft, but not mushy. As the beans cook add other ingredients called for in the recipe and add liquid as it cooks down. Add salt, herbs, and spices in the last 20 minutes. Smaller beans such as lentils and green peas require less cooking time. Follow the package directions.

APPETIZER

Pears with Black Pepper and Blue Cheese

This is a simple, knockout dish to serve before dinner, as a side dish, or just to indulge yourself. All you do is sprinkle crumbled blue cheese or feta cheese over fresh sliced pears.

Serves 2

INGREDIENTS

1 firm, ripe pear, such as Bosc

Black pepper, to taste

⅓ cup crumbled blue cheese or feta cheese

METHOD

1. Slice the pear in quarters and remove the core and stem. Peeling is not necessary. Cut each quarter in half so you have 8 pieces.

2. Arrange the pear pieces on a plate. Sprinkle the pear slices with the black pepper and then the crumbled cheese. Serve on small plates and eat with a fork.

SALAD

Cherry or Grape Tomato Salad

Serves 2

INGREDIENTS

10 cherry or grape tomatoes

1-2 teaspoons bottled low-fat, low-salt salad dressing such as Italian or Caesar or Homemade Salad Dressing, recipe page 83

Salt and pepper to taste

METHOD

Wash tomatoes, halve, and place 10 halves on each of two small plates. Sprinkle about a teaspoon of the salad dressing over the tomatoes. Add salt and pepper, if necessary. Refrigerate leftover salad dressing.

ENTREES

LIGHT MEALS

SUPER EASY

Quick Marinara Spaghetti Sauce

"This is good!" Jean Wilson

The ingredient list may seem long, but this dish is very easy to cook. Make a large pot or saucepan of this recipe and keep the leftovers in the freezer for many other dishes besides spaghetti and pastas.

INGREDIENTS

1 tablespoon extra virgin olive oil or canola oil

2 teaspoons onion powder or minced onion, or ½ small onion, peeled and chopped3 teaspoons powdered garlic or minced dried garlic, or 2 cloves fresh garlic, peeled and chopped

¾ cup pre-washed packaged fresh bell pepper or fresh chopped bell pepper

2 cans 14.5-ounce diced tomatoes, your choice of flavor, salt free if available

1 14.5-ounce can tomato sauce, salt free if available

2 teaspoons dried basil or ½ cup fresh basil, chopped

2 teaspoons dried oregano or ½ cup fresh oregano leaves

Salt and pepper to taste

227

METHOD

1. Heat oil in a medium to large saucepan. If using fresh onion, add chopped onion to heated saucepan and sauté till translucent. Add chopped bell pepper to the pan and sauté for about 2 to 4 minutes. Add chopped fresh garlic last and cook about 1 minute.

2. Add the cans of diced tomatoes and the tomato sauce to the pot or saucepan. Stir until the sauce is thoroughly mixed.

3. At this time, add powdered or dried onion and garlic along with the basil and oregano. Stir again. Taste and adjust the seasonings, adding more herbs and salt and pepper, according to your taste.fre

4. Bring the sauce to a boil, stirring occasionally. When the sauce begins to boil, turn the heat down immediately so the sauce simmers for about two hours. Taste and adjust the seasonings again.

5. Serve over pasta, in lasagna, soups, stews, over meats, or in other dishes as desired. Reserve leftover sauce in containers and place in the freezer for future use.

Recipe tested by Jean Wilson

Meat Spaghetti Sauce

The marinara spaghetti sauce recipe can easily be turned into a meat sauce by adding ½ pound lean ground meat, either beef, pork, chicken, or turkey. Add it to the sautéing fresh onion, garlic, and bell pepper. Crumble the ground meat with a wooden spoon. Then continue with the recipe above recipe.

Pretty Dang Tasty Cabbage

"I will make this dish again!" Kathy Cain Parkins

Serves 4-6

INGREDIENTS

- 1-2 teaspoons extra virgin olive oil or canola oil, as needed

- 1 teaspoon powdered or minced dried onion; 1 cup scallions, roots and browned leaves removed; or onion of your choice, chopped

- 2 teaspoons powdered or minced dried garlic, or 3-4 cloves garlic, peeled and chopped

- 1 4-ounce can diced chili peppers, mild, or 1 banana chili pepper, split open, seeded, and chopped

- 1 tablespoon sesame seeds, optional

- 3 cups packaged, diced, pre-washed cabbage or ½ small head of cabbage, finely sliced

- ½ cup vegetable or chicken broth, low-salt and reduced-fat, or white wine

- 1 whole fresh tomato, chopped, or 1 14.5 ounce can diced tomato, drained, your choice of flavors

- 1 cup chopped, cooked chicken breast or 1 block firm tofu, cubed (Available in fresh produce section) or boxed aseptic tofu (in Japanese food section.) The tofu is optional.

METHOD

1. On a medium-to-high setting, heat the oil in a large skillet. Add scallions or onions and garlic, if using fresh, chili peppers, and sesame seeds, if using. Stir for about 30 seconds. Remove from heat if necessary to prevent burning.

2. Add sliced cabbage and stir to mix. At this time, add dried onion and garlic, if using.

3. Stir. Pour in broth or wine and stir. Reduce heat to low, and add tomato. Cover.

4. Simmer until cabbage reaches desired tenderness, 5 to 10 minutes. Add more broth if the mixture becomes dry. Add chopped chicken or tofu, if using, to warm.

5. Adapted from a Wellspring (now Whole Foods) flyer, Durham, North Carolina, 1997

Recipe tested by Kathy Cain Parkins

Crustless Quiche: Spinach, Bell Pepper, and Feta or Parmesan

"This is a good recipe." Linda Prospero

Serves 4-6

INGREDIENTS

1 tablespoon extra virgin olive oil or canola oil

½ cup pre-washed packaged bell pepper, or chopped bell pepper, seeds and pith removed

1 teaspoon powdered or dried minced onion or 1 cup fresh onion, chopped finely

1 box frozen spinach, defrosted and moisture removed by squeezing or 1 pre-washed package fresh baby spinach leaves

1 teaspoon dried basil or 10 fresh basil leaves, chopped

Salt and pepper to taste, adding a minimum

½ cup low-fat or skim milk or "milk" of your choice, not sweet

4 eggs

½ cup crumbled feta cheese or shredded Parmesan

METHOD

1. Preheat oven to 400 degrees. Grease bottom of pie plate or baking pan with 1 to 2 teaspoons oil.

2. Quarter and remove the pith and seeds of the bell pepper. Chop the bell pepper and onion, if using fresh.

3. Add 1 to 2 teaspoons oil to a large, non-stick skillet over medium high heat. Sauté bell pepper, stirring, for about 1 minute, and then add the chopped onion and sauté until translucent.

4. Remove water from the defrosted frozen spinach by squeezing with your hands. If using fresh baby spinach, wash and pat dry with paper towels. Add spinach to the skillet with the other vegetables, if using, stirring for 1 to 2 minutes, until well mixed.

5. If using powdered or dried onion and garlic, add to the skillet at this point. Stir.

6. Remove skillet from heat and season bell pepper, onion, and spinach mixture with basil, salt, and pepper to your taste. Stir.

7. In a small bowl, stir together eggs and milk or "milk" of your choice (not a sweet milk).

8. Sprinkle feta or Parmesan cheese over bottom of oiled pie plate or baking pan. Arrange vegetable and spinach mixture on top of cheese. Pour egg mixture over spinach and bake crustless quiche in middle of oven for 20 to 25 minutes.

9. Test for doneness by inserting a sharp knife in the middle. If it comes out clean, the crustless quiche is ready. Wait about 10 minutes and then slice into serving-size pieces. Serve with a salad on the side and warmed whole wheat baguette.

Recipe tested by Linda Prospero

BEAN DISHES

Lentil, Chickpea, and Vegetable Stew
Serves 4-6

INGREDIENTS

- 1 tablespoon extra virgin olive oil or canola oil
- 2 teaspoons powdered or dried minced onion or 1 onion, peeled and chopped
- 2 teaspoons powdered or dried minced garlic or 3 garlic cloves, peeled and chopped
- 1 4-ounce can tomato paste
- 2 teaspoons ground coriander, optional
- 1 teaspoon caraway seeds, optional
- Pinch of cayenne pepper, optional
- ½ 16-ounce package dried lentils
- Low-fat, low-salt vegetable or chicken broth and water to cover the uncooked lentils by ½ to 1 inch
- 1 15-ounce can chickpeas, rinsed and drained
- 1 cup pre-washed packaged chopped or slivered carrots or 10 baby carrots, halved or 2 medium carrots, peeled and sliced thinly
- 1 bag or box frozen lima beans
- 2 teaspoons dried parsley or ½ cup chopped parsley
- 1 box frozen spinach with no added fats or sugar, defrosted and squeezed dry, or 1 cup fresh baby spinach

METHOD

1. Add oil to a large pot or saucepan over medium heat. If using fresh onion and garlic, add to the pot or saucepan. Cook until onions are translucent, for 2 to 5 minutes.

2. Add the tomato paste and spices, if using, and stir until mixed. Add powdered or dried minced onion and garlic at this time.

3. Stir in dried lentils, broth and water or a mix. Increase heat to high and bring to a boil. Immediately reduce the heat, cover, and simmer until lentils are almost tender, stirring occasionally, for 15 to 25 minutes.

4. Add canned chickpeas, carrots, lima beans, and the parsley. Cover; simmer until carrots are very tender, about 20 minutes.

5. If using fresh spinach, stir into the stew in batches until wilted. Or add the defrosted and squeezed-dry spinach.

6. Season with salt and pepper to taste. Ladle into bowls with cooked brown rice, recipe page 86.

SUPER EASY

Red Bean Soup

"Taste the flavors of New Orleans in this easy and flavorful soup. I'm surprised at how quick this dish is, especially if you use canned red beans." Ruth Porter

Serves 4-6

INGREDIENTS

1 tablespoon extra virgin olive oil or canola oil

1 teaspoon onion powder or dried minced onion or
1 cup onions, chopped

1 stalk celery, chopped, optional

½ cup pre-washed packaged bell pepper, or bell pepper that is seeded, pith removed, and chopped

2 bay leaves, optional

2 teaspoons dried cilantro or
½ cup fresh cilantro, chopped, optional

½ teaspoon cayenne pepper, optional

**1 teaspoon powdered or dried minced garlic or
2 cloves garlic, peeled and chopped**

**2 15.5-ounce cans red beans, rinsed and drained, or
3 cups cooked dry red beans, recipe page 225**

**1 box or 2 cans vegetarian or chicken broth, with
little or no salt or fat, plus water**

**1 tablespoon bottled pure lemon juice or juice of
1 lemon or 1 tablespoon vinegar**

METHOD

1. Heat oil in a large pot or saucepan over medium heat. If using fresh onions, add to the heated oil and cook until the onions are translucent.

2. Add the celery, bell pepper, bay leaves, and cayenne, if using, and cook until the vegetables are just beginning to brown and are very tender, about 5 minutes. Add fresh garlic, if using, and stir for about 30 seconds.

3. At this time, add powdered or dried minced onion and garlic, if using.

4. Stir and immediately add red beans and broth and water. Bring to a boil. Reduce the heat and simmer uncovered, stirring occasionally, for about 20 minutes.

5. Using an immersion or handheld blender or the back of a fork, mash some of the beans slightly to thicken the broth. Continue cooking uncovered for about another 10 minutes, or until the soup has thickened.

6. Remove from the heat and discard the bay leaves, if using. Serve hot with brown rice, whole grain bread, or corn bread.

Recipe tested by Ruth Porter

CHICKEN RECIPES

Chicken Salad with Celery and Walnuts

Excellent for use of leftover chicken breast.

Serves 2-4

INGREDIENTS

1-2 cups cooked, leftover chicken breast, cut into bite-size pieces

1 cup celery, sliced into ½ inch pieces, or from pre-washed packaged celery

1 stalk green onions, roots cut off and sliced into ½ inch pieces, or ½ cup onion, chopped

Handful of roasted walnuts, chopped

1 tablespoon lite mayonnaise

1 tablespoon nonfat plain yogurt or Greek yogurt

1 teaspoon dried tarragon

Juice of 1 lemon or 1 tablespoon bottled pure lemon juice or vinegar

1 teaspoon dried parsley or ¼ cup fresh parsley, chopped

Salt and pepper to taste, using minimum

Lettuce leaves for serving

Tomato wedges for serving

METHOD

1. Roast walnuts (recipe page 149) and chop.

2. Cut chicken breast into bite-size pieces.

3. Put chicken, celery, onions, lite mayonnaise, yogurt, walnuts, and salt and pepper into a medium-size bowl. Toss until combined.

4. Refrigerate for 1 to 2 hours to cool, if possible. Place lettuce leaves on serving plates with tomato wedges.

Oven-Fried Chicken

You've heard of this, and now you know how to make this healthy version of a Southern favorite. There are three basic steps: Marinating in buttermilk, coating in self-rising flour, and baking. Now that's easy!

Adapted from Paula Deen on Dr. Oz.

Serves 4-6

INGREDIENTS

Marinade

> 1 cup nonfat buttermilk (Try to keep buttermilk on hand. Use it as a tenderizer for chicken and as well as in making cornbread, pancakes, and other baked goods.)
>
> 1 teaspoon garlic powder or dried minced garlic
>
> Salt and pepper, to taste, keeping salt to a minimum
>
> 2 chicken breasts, cut into 4 to 6 pieces, or 4 chicken thighs, boneless and skinless, trimmed of fat

Breading

> 1 cup self-rising flour, whole wheat if available
>
> Salt and pepper, to taste, keeping salt to a minimum

METHOD

1. Plan ahead so you have time to soak the chicken in the buttermilk.

2. Cut the chicken into serving-size pieces. Place them in a gallon, zippered, heavy plastic bag. In a bowl or large measuring cup, stir the buttermilk, garlic, salt, and pepper together. Pour the buttermilk marinade into the bag with the chicken. Seal, turn to coat all the pieces of chicken, and place in the refrigerator for at 1 to 2 hours.

3. When you are ready to bake the chicken pieces, preheat oven to 450 degrees. Cover a rimmed cookie sheet or line a large baking pan with aluminum foil. Place a rack in the bottom of the pan.

4. Put the self-rising flour and salt and pepper, to taste, into a clean, zippered, heavy plastic bag.

5. Remove chicken pieces from the buttermilk marinade bag. Allow the excess moisture from the chicken to drain over the sink or into a bowl.

6. Add 1 or 2 drained chicken pieces at a time to the bag with the flour, and when you do, zip the bag closed and shake it so each piece is thoroughly covered with the flour. Place the flour-covered chicken pieces on a rack on the cookie sheet or baking pan. This raises the chicken off the bottom.

7. Do not overlap the pieces but allow air space between each piece. Bake for 40 to 50 minutes or until the chicken is golden brown and when pressed the juices run clear, not pink.

8. Enjoy! Serve with salad and bread of your choice.

Chicken Cacciatore, Italian-American Style

"Overall, a very tasty dish, easy to make, and I'm sure I will make it again for friends." Ann Hall

This is my late mother-in-law's recipe.

Serves 4-6

INGREDIENTS

1-3 tablespoons extra virgin olive oil or canola oil

2 teaspoons powdered or dried minced garlic or 3 cloves fresh garlic, peeled and chopped

1 teaspoon powdered or minced dried onion or 1 small onion, peeled and chopped

1 cup pre-washed packaged bell pepper or 1 cup bell pepper, seeds and pith removed, chopped

2-4 chicken breasts, boneless and skinless, 1 pound boneless and skinless chicken thighs, or combination

½ cup pimento-stuffed green olives, sliced in half

1 28-ounce can whole tomatoes

1 teaspoon dried oregano

1 teaspoon dried basil or ½ cup fresh basil, chopped

Salt and pepper, to taste, adding a minimum of salt

METHOD

1. In a heavy skillet on medium heat, place enough oil, 1 to 3 tablespoons, to sauté fresh garlic and onion, if using, until onion is translucent. Add chopped bell pepper and cook until barely limp.

2. Move vegetables to the side and add chicken pieces. Brown lightly on both sides.

3. Slice or chop tomatoes in a bowl. Add olives, chopped whole tomatoes, oregano, and basil. Adjust all seasonings to taste, adding at this time the powdered and dried minced onion and garlic, if using.

4. Cover. Simmer for about 20 to 30 minutes or until chicken is done. Serve with brown rice, recipe page 80.

Recipe tested by Ann Hall

Sautéed Chicken or Pork Chops with Apples

"We liked this a lot!" Ruth Porter

This is a good dish for fall or winter, and like so many others, easy, simple, and cheap.

Serves 2-4

INGREDIENTS

1 tablespoon extra virgin olive oil or canola oil

2 whole skinless, boneless chicken breasts or 4-6 skinless, boneless chicken thighs or 4 thin, boneless pork chops, trimmed of fat

1 teaspoon powdered or dried minced onion or 1 small onion, peeled and chopped

1 apple, such as Granny Smith, delicious, or gala, quartered, cored, peeled, and sliced or 1 cup dried apple slices

1 tablespoon apple cider vinegar or white vinegar

½ cup apple cider or apple juice (Can be from individual drink cartons.)

Salt and pepper, to taste, keeping salt to a minimum

METHOD

1. **Chicken:** Trim fat off all of the chicken. Divide breast into 3 to 4 pieces and lightly sprinkle pepper over front and back of chicken. Flatten by covering with Saran Wrap and pounding with the rounded side of a can or mallet.

2. Heat oil in a large nonstick skillet. Add chicken and sauté until browned, about 5 minutes per side. Remove chicken from the skillet.

3. Add fresh onion to the skillet and cook until translucent and softened, about 3-4 minutes. Add fresh apple slices, if using, to the skillet sautéing for about 2 minutes. At this time, add powdered or dried minced onion to the skillet and stir.

4. Return the chicken to the pan, adding the vinegar and juice. Simmer until no pink liquid comes from the chicken when pressed.

5. Remove the chicken pieces to a platter and pour remaining juice into a bowl. Serve the chicken with brown rice (recipe page 80) and a salad. Use the juice to moisten the chicken and rice.

6. **Pork chops:** Follow the above directions, substituting the pork chops for the chicken and reducing the cooking time to 3 minutes per side. Do not flatten by pounding or cut into smaller pieces. Pork chops go well with apple.

Recipe tested by Ruth Porter

GROUND MEAT

Picadillo *Puerto Rican*

"The picadillo was very tasty. I love the flavor of the cumin and the pimientos." Ann Hall

Picadillo *means chopped or minced. A Puerto Rican lady gave me this recipe many years ago. She often used fried ripe plantains with it, but that's not included in this recipe. The important ingredients are, besides the ground beef, the olives and raisins, salty and sweet, along with the herbs and spices. Serve with brown rice and beans of your choice. Black beans are most often used in Puerto Rico.*

Serves 4-6

INGREDIENTS

1 tablespoon extra virgin olive oil or canola oil

2 teaspoons powdered or dried minced onion or
½ to 1 cup fresh onion, chopped

1 cup pre-washed packaged bell pepper, chopped, or
1 prepared fresh bell pepper

1 teaspoon garlic powder or dried minced garlic or
1 clove garlic, chopped

1 teaspoon dried oregano

1 pound 93-96 % lean ground beef

½ cup olives stuffed with pimientos, halved

240

½ to ¾ cup raisins

½ teaspoon ground cumin, use this if possible

½ teaspoon ground cinnamon, optional

1 8-ounce can tomato sauce or
    4 ounce can tomato paste

Salt and pepper to taste, using a minimum

1 box frozen French-style green beans, optional

METHOD

1. Heat oil on medium heat on the stovetop in a large non-stick or cast iron skillet. Add fresh chopped onion, if using, and bell pepper and cook until the onion is translucent and the bell pepper is tender. Add the fresh garlic, if using, and oregano. Stir until well blended.

2. Add the ground beef and with the back of a wooden spoon spread the meat in the pan until it is in small bits and cooked through. Add the powdered or dried onion and garlic, at this time, cumin and cinnamon, if using, olives, and raisins. Mix well.

3. Add the tomato sauce or paste and combine until the tomato sauce or paste is mixed throughout. Add ¼ to ½ cup liquid, such as broth or wine, as necessary to combine easily.

4. Taste and adjust seasonings, adding salt and pepper if necessary.

5. Continue to cook on low heat for about 10 minutes. When ready to serve, place the *picadillo* in a serving dish and top with the optional cooked French-style green beans. Serve with brown rice and beans on the side.

Recipe tested by Ann Hall

Classic Meatloaf

This is the recipe I grew up making, and it's moist, tasty, and healthy, too.

Serves 4-6

INGREDIENTS

> 1 pound 93-96% lean ground beef or ground lean turkey
>
> 2 teaspoons powdered or dried minced onion or ½-¾ cup onion, finely chopped
>
> 1 egg
>
> ½ cup canned tomato sauce
>
> 1 cup uncooked quick or regular oatmeal
>
> Salt and pepper, to taste, keeping salt to a minimum
>
> 1 teaspoon oregano, dried
>
> 1 teaspoon basil, dried
>
> 1 tablespoon extra virgin olive oil or canola oil
>
> Salt and pepper to taste
>
> 2 tablespoons ketchup

METHOD

1. Preheat oven to 350 degrees.

2. Place ground meat in a medium-size bowl. Add onion, egg, tomato sauce, dry oats, oregano, basil, 2 teaspoons oil, and salt and pepper to taste. Blend completely with a spoon or your hands.

3. Grease a loaf pan with remaining oil and shape the meat mixture into a loaf. Place the meat mixture into the pan and spread the ketchup on top. Place on a middle rack in the oven and bake at 350 degrees for 65 minutes or so.

4. Remove from the oven and let rest for about 10 minutes. Slice the meatloaf in the pan and serve with brown rice (recipe page 80) and a salad or vegetable, such as green beans (recipe page 210).

FISH

Summer Tuna Fish Salad for Two

"It's really delicious and works both as a salad or sandwich filling. Terrific lunch on a hot day with a glass of iced tea." Carol Wills

Serves 2

INGREDIENTS

- 2 6.4-ounce packets or cans dark meat tuna packed in water
- 1 pre-washed packaged celery or 1 stalk celery, chopped
- 1 teaspoon powdered or dried minced onion or ½ cup onion, chopped
- 1 apple, such as gala, Granny Smith, delicious, seeded and cut into pieces about the size of the celery
- Juice of 1 lemon or 1 tablespoon bottled pure lemon juice or 2 teaspoons vinegar
- 2 teaspoons lite mayonnaise
- 2 teaspoons plain or Greek yogurt, low-fat or fat-free
- 4 whole lettuce leaves, washed and drained
- Salt to taste

METHOD

1. Combine tuna, onion, celery, and apple and toss. Pour lemon juice or vinegar over ingredients. Toss.

2. Add mayonnaise and yogurt and toss until all ingredients are well combined. Serve over lettuce leaves spread on plates. Season with salt, to taste. Offer crackers or pita bread to accompany.

3. This dish can also be made without the mayonnaise and yogurt.

Recipe tested by Carol Wills

So Easy Salmon Fillet Bake with Lemon

If you don't feel like cooking or mixing up a sauce, but you are determined to stay healthy, this recipe's for you. All you need, beside the salmon fillet, is some oil and lemon. That's it, and you've got a delicious dinner.

Serves 4-6

INGREDIENTS

1 pound salmon fillet, cut from the thick end

1 tablespoon extra virgin olive oil or canola oil

Zest and juice from 1 lemon or
1 tablespoon bottled pure lemon juice or vinegar of your choice

Salt and pepper to taste

METHOD

1. Preheat oven to 350 degrees. Cover a rimmed cookie sheet with aluminum foil.

2. If using fresh lemon, zest the yellow part of a lemon by scraping on the smallest grates of a handheld grater. Sprinkle the zest over the salmon. (This step is optional, but it adds a real zing to the flavor.) Squeeze the juice from the lemon over the salmon's skinless side, removing any seeds that have fallen.

3. If not using fresh lemon, pour bottled lemon juice or vinegar over the fillet.

4. Place the cookie sheet with the salmon, prepared side up and skin side down, in the middle of the oven and bake for 20 to 25 minutes. The flesh should be opaque and flaky when the fish is done.

5. Remove from the oven and while the fish is still on the cookie sheet, turn the fillet over, and scrape the skin off and discard.

6. Cut into serving-size pieces and place on plates or a platter. Serve with brown rice and salad. Spoon any sauce from the pan over the fish and rice.

Baked Tilapia with Spinach

This recipe combines the white-fleshed tilapia fish with vegetables, making a complete meal with some added brown rice.

Serves 4-6

INGREDIENTS

2-4 small tilapia fillets, either fresh or flash-frozen, not flavored

1 tablespoon extra virgin olive oil or canola oil

1 box or bag frozen spinach or 1 package fresh pre-washed baby spinach leaves

¼ cup chicken or vegetarian broth, in a box or can, reduced-fat and low-salt, or white wine

¼ teaspoon onion powder or dried minced onion, or ½ cup onion, chopped

1 small tomato, chopped, or 4 grape or cherry tomatoes, halved

Salt and pepper, to taste, using a minimum of salt

METHOD

1. Pre-heat the oven to 350 degrees. Oil a baking dish large enough to fit the fish fillets in it.

2. In making this dish, you will add the broth or wine to the baking dish. If using fresh spinach, add the spinach leaves, pushing them down to fit into the baking dish. As the dish bakes, they will fit the dish.

3. If using frozen spinach, allow it to thaw for 2 to 3 hours before beginning to cook. With your hands, squeeze out the excess moisture. Place the thawed spinach in the bottom of the oiled baking dish.

4. Place the fillets on top of the spinach and then the tomatoes and onion over the fillets.

5. Cover the baking dish with foil and bake at 350° for 20 to 25 minutes, or until fish flakes easily with a fork.

6. Serve the tilapia and spinach with brown rice as a side.

SOUPS

Easy Soup, Basic Recipe
4-6 servings

INGREDIENTS

4-6 cups canned or boxed broth, low-salt and low-fat

1 14.5-ounce can tomatoes, diced, any flavor

1 cup pre-washed packaged celery or 1 stalk celery, chopped, including leaves

1-2 tablespoons uncooked brown rice, barley, or bulgur wheat

¼ teaspoon hot sauce, or to taste, optional

1-2 teaspoons dried herbs such as thyme, oregano, basil, or your choice

2 teaspoon dried parsley or 1 tablespoon fresh parsley, chopped

2 teaspoons onion powder

½ cup frozen or canned lima beans, rinsed to remove excess salt

1 box or bag, frozen mixed vegetables, small or large

Salt and pepper, to taste

½ to 1 cup leftover chicken, chopped

(You can add chopped vegetables or other cooked meat that you have on hand.)

METHOD

1. Add all ingredients except cooked chicken to a large pot or saucepan. Simmer for 1 hour or until vegetables are tender.

2. Taste soup as it cooks and adjust seasoning as needed, adding more broth, onion powder, dried herbs, or salt and pepper to taste. Keep salt to a minimum.

3. Add cooked chicken or other chopped meat and continue cooking for 10 more minutes.

4. Serve with warmed, leftover cornbread or whole wheat bread or crackers.

SUPER EASY

Easy Lentil Soup with Vegetables
Serves 4

INGREDIENTS

1 16-ounce package of dried lentil beans

1 tablespoon extra virgin olive oil or canola oil

1 teaspoon onion powder or dried minced onion or
½ cup onion, chopped

1 teaspoon powdered or dried minced garlic or
1 clove garlic, peeled and chopped

½ cup pre-washed, packaged shredded carrots,
4-6 baby carrots, sliced, or 1 whole carrot,
washed, scraped, and sliced

½ cup pre-washed, packaged bell pepper or
¼ bell pepper, seeded, pith removed, and chopped

1 carton or 2 cans vegetarian or chicken broth,
low-salt and reduced-fat

Water—enough to cover lentils in addition to the
broth about 1 inch in the saucepan

1-2 teaspoons dried thyme, or dried herb of your
choice

Salt and pepper, to taste

METHOD

1. Pour lentils into a colander and remove any stones or misshapen lentils. Rinse thoroughly until water runs clear.

2. Heat oil over medium heat in a large pot or saucepan. Add fresh onions and garlic, if using, carrots, and bell pepper and sauté until tender and just brown.

3. Add lentils and stir till the vegetables and lentils are mixed. At this time, add herb(s) and powdered or dried minced onion and garlic, if using. Stir all ingredients to mix well.

4. Immediately, pour broth and water into pot or saucepan to cover lentils about 1 inch (add more water as the lentils are cooking if necessary) and over high heat bring to a rolling boil.

5. After the liquid comes to a boil, turn down the heat so the soup simmers. Cover and allow to simmer for 1 ½ to 2 hours, or more as needed, till the lentils are tender, but not mushy. Add salt and pepper in the last 20 minutes. Taste and adjust seasonings.

6. Serve in bowls with brown rice or couscous, recipes pages 80-81, and cornbread, recipe page 134.

SIDES

Pan-Cooked Brussels Sprouts with Garlic
Serves 4-6

INGREDIENTS

1 tablespoon extra virgin olive oil or canola oil

1 pound Brussels sprouts, ends trimmed, yellowed leaves removed, and cut into quarters

1 teaspoon powdered or dried minced garlic or 2 cloves garlic, peeled and chopped

Salt and pepper, to taste, kept to a minimum

1 teaspoon dried parsley or 1 tablespoon fresh parsley, chopped

Method

1. Heat the oil in a large, non-stick skillet over medium-high heat.

2. Add the prepared Brussels sprouts. Cook, tossing gently, until they begin to color, about 5 minutes.

3. Turn down the heat to medium and add the garlic. Continue to cook, stirring, until the Brussels sprouts are tender, another 3 to 5 minutes.

4. Stir in the parsley and salt and pepper to taste, and adjust seasonings if necessary. Serve as a side dish to a roast.

Super Easy

Asparagus with Creamy Tarragon Sauce

This sauce is creamy and delicious without all the calories and fat.

Serves 4-6

INGREDIENTS

2 bunches fresh asparagus, tough ends trimmed, or
   1 box frozen asparagus, with little or no fat or
   sugar added, or 2 cans asparagus

½ cup low-fat or fat-free plain yogurt

3 tablespoons lite mayonnaise

1 teaspoon dried tarragon

Juice from 1 lemon or 1 tablespoon bottled pure
   lemon juice or 1 teaspoon vinegar

1 tablespoon water

1 teaspoon Dijon mustard

Salt and pepper to taste, salt kept to a minimum

METHOD

1. Prepare the tarragon sauce first so it's ready when the asparagus is. Whisk or beat with a fork the yogurt, mayonnaise, tarragon, lemon juice or vinegar, water, mustard, salt and pepper in a small bowl. Reserve till the asparagus is ready to serve.

2. If using fresh asparagus, hold each stalk of the fresh asparagus by the flower end. With the other hand, bend the stalk and snap off the tough part.

3. Cook by adding water to just below the base of a steamer basket and laying asparagus in the basket. Cover the saucepan and steam until tender-crisp, about 4 minutes.

4. If using frozen asparagus, follow package directions. If using canned, drain and rinse to wash off excess salt. Warm in a saucepan or in microwave very gently.

5. When heated and ready to serve, place on a serving plate and drizzle tarragon sauce over the asparagus.

Sweet Potato Circles

Serves 2-4

INGREDIENTS

1-2 sweet potatoes

1 tablespoon extra virgin olive oil or canola oil

1 tablespoon light brown sugar

METHOD

1. Thoroughly wash and scrub the sweet potatoes. Peel, if desired. (You can eat the washed peel.) Slice across the long part of the sweet potatoes, making circles.

2. Coat the slices with oil and spread them in a single layer on an aluminum-foil-lined rimmed cookie sheet.

3. Sprinkle lightly with the brown sugar and bake for about 30 minutes until tender and beginning to brown. Remove from oven and serve.

Recipe from Carol Wills

DESSERTS

Peaches with Yogurt
Serves 2

INGREDIENTS

1 14.5 can peaches; 1 package frozen peach slices, no sugar added; or 1 fresh peach, ripe

2 tablespoons vanilla yogurt, or vanilla Greek yogurt

METHOD

1. If using a fresh peach, cut into small, bite-size pieces, discarding the pit. If you prefer, peel the peach first. If using canned or frozen, drain the peaches and cut into bite-sized pieces.

2. Place ½ cup peaches into each of 2 small bowls and top with vanilla yogurt. Reserve any remaining peaches in a plastic container in the refrigerator for future use.

3. Serve for dessert, breakfast, or a snack with milk.

Chilled Strawberry Soup

This easy dessert is a surprise because it's so creamy and yet so healthy. There's no cooking and all you need is a stand-alone blender or an immersion or handheld blender, or even a food processor.

Serves 4-6

INGREDIENTS

> **1 pound fresh strawberries, washed, stems removed, and quartered, or 1 box or bag frozen strawberries with no added sugar**
>
> **2 tablespoons low-fat sour cream or low-fat or fat-free plain yogurt**
>
> **2 cups low-fat or skim milk, "milk," or fat-free half-and-half**
>
> **1 tablespoon brown sugar or honey, or to taste**

METHOD

1. Place washed and prepared strawberries in the bowl of a food processor, blender, or immersion or handheld blender. Puree until the strawberries are smooth and almost liquid.

2. Add sour cream or yogurt; milk, "milk," or fat-free half-and-half; and brown sugar or honey. Thoroughly blend until all the ingredients are mixed.

3. Pour the "soup" into a sealed container or jar and chill in the refrigerator for at least two hours before serving.

4. Serve in small cups or bowls with a quarter of a low-fat graham cracker on the side. Strawberry Soup may be drunk or eaten with a spoon.

Chapter 17

Keep Going

Finding More Information

Here are suggestions to get you started on your search for more information on a healthy lifestyle. As you begin your search, you will find other sources. It's an adventure. But be careful. Many of the sites and publications are unreliable. If it's too easy, be wary.

Information on the Web

HEALTHY LIFESTYLE, HEALTHY EATING, AND EXERCISE

Food Network, www.foodnetwork.com/healthy-eating/index.html

About.com This web site has a great deal of information. Try the following links for more information on health and cooking when you're busy:

> about.com/health

> busycooks.about.com

WebMD The following link has good information on food, recipes, and weight loss:

> http://www.webmd.com/food-recipes/default.htm

For information on fitness and exercise, go to:

> www.webmd.com/fitness-exercise/guide/

Government Publications

WEIGHT CONTROL AND HEALTHY LIVING

The following government publications are free:

The Weight-Control Information Network (WIN)

> http://win.niddk.nih.gov/publications/index.htm#public

Centers for Disease Control and Prevention

> http://www.cdc.gov/healthyweight/index.html

MedLine Plus

> http://www.nlm.nih.gov/medlineplus

ABOUT EXERCISE

These free government booklets are excellent to have on hand for reference and to use:

> http://catalog.gpo.gov Type into the search space: Exercise and Physical Activity
>
> http://www.weboflife.nasa.gov/exerciseandaging/toc.html.

Other Sources of Information on the Web

Center for Science in the Public Interest. This site is an excellent source of current food policy and information:

> http://cspinet.org/nutritionpolicy/

Siteman Cancer Center, Washington University School of Medicine, promotes healthy living for avoiding common diseases:

http://www.yourdeseaserisk.wustl.edu

Magazines

MAGAZINES, PRINT OR ONLINE

Cooking Light   http://www.cookinglight.com. Information on nutrition, super fast recipes, and more.

Eating Well   http://www.eatingwell.com. There you can subscribe to several newsletters.

Fitness   http://www.fitnessmagazine.com Geared toward the 20-something age group, it takes some searching but you can find healthy and quick recipes.

Health   http://www.health.com The recipes are somewhat involved, but it's good reading.

Self   http://self.com Like *Fitness,* this magazine is geared toward the 20-something crowd. But you can find some good recipes and shortcuts.

Books

PRINT AND E-BOOKS

Hanh, Thich Nhat, and Lian Cheung.   *Savor: Mindful Eating, Mindful Life.* San Francisco: HarperCollins, 2010. A Zen Buddhist approach to a healthy life and healthy eating.

Katzen, Mollie and Walter C. Willett.   *Eat, Drink, & Weigh Less: A Flexible and Delicious Way to Shrink Your Waist Without Going Hungry.* New York: Hyperion. 2007. Written by cookbook author Mollie Katzen and head of Harvard School of Public Health.

Willett, Walter C., and P.J. Skerrett. *Eat, Drink, and Be Healthy: The Harvard Medical School Guide to Healthy Eating.* Free Press. 2007, Kindle ed., 2011. Reflects current research on healthy nutrition by head of Harvard School of Public Health. Very helpful in understanding nutrition for a healthy life.

Vegetarian Books

PRINT AND E-BOOKS

Del Stroufe, Julieanna Hever, Isa Chandra Moskowitz, and Darshana Thacker. *Forks over Knives: The Cookbook,* The Experiment: New York, 2012.

Furham, Joel. *Eat to Live: The Amazing Nutrient-Rich Program for Fast and Sustained Weight Loss.* Rev. Ed. New York: Little, Brown and Company, 2012.

Esselstyn, Rip. *The Engine 2 Diet: The Texas Firefighter's 28-Day Save-Your-Life Plan that Lowers Cholesterol and Burns Away the Pounds.* New York: Grand Central Life & Style, 2009.

Stone, Gene, Colin T. Campbell, and Caldwell Esselstyn, Jr. *Forks over Knives: The Plant Based Way to Health.* The Experiment: New York, 2011.

Chapter 18

Afterword

George W. Newton

On Healthy Eating

Georgge W. Newton inspired me to write this book by first asking for a meal plan for seniors, then envisioning it as an aid to all who are struggling to become and remain healthy, especially to the growing number of obese individuals.

As a creative and successful engineer, founder of the Newton Instrument Company, and founding trustee of Durham Tech Community College, first known as Durham Instrument Education Center, George turned his creativity to health, seeking to benefit all those who don't know how to be healthy or who think health is out of their reach.

To achieve this goal, he devised the "Healthy Eating Plan," based on on six days of menus for the spring/summer and fall/winter seasons, as a means of beginning and staying on a healthy life plan. He writes of this plan below:

"The most important parts of your daily life are the meals that you consume. Your diet largely controls your short-term and long-term well being.

"To plan, shop, and prepare meals is a time-consuming task. The menus presented in the 'Healthy Eating Plan' are balanced and include simple, healthy recipes and menus. To accommodate seasonal foods, there are two standard menus, one for Spring and Summer and one for Fall and Winter. There are also chapters on celebration menus and recipes and on additional menus and recipes.

"Why a six-day cycle? Eighteen meals in each season for breakfast, lunch, and dinner, as well as for snacks, include most of the foods commonly needed in the average diet. By having a six-day rotation, you avoid having the same meal appear every Tuesday, for example. The plan works best if you stay with the cycle even though an event may interrupt it. Continue with the plan as soon as possible as though there has not been an interruption. You will find the plan flexible enough to satisfy most tastes as well as meet special diet requirements."

George W. Newton

Recipe Index

The Author

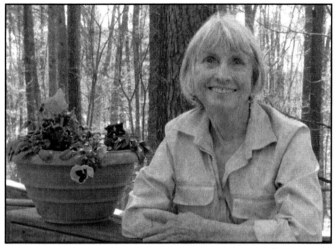

Photo: John H. Fricks

Ann Prospero has spent a lifetime living the principles of healthy living and four years researching and writing her book, *Even You Can Be Healthy!* A professional woman who also raised a family, she knows first hand that we lead busy, stressed, and sometimes economically challenged lives. As a consequence, she simplifies the three steps—exercise, calming, and healthy eating—that will lead to a healthy life.

Prospero spent four years investigating these subjects for her book, *Even You Can Be Healthy!* Throughout her professional career, she wrote, researched, and edited numerous articles and publications for local, regional, and national outlets. She has dealt with subjects that range from horticulture to spirituality to football. Dutton in New York and four publishers in Europe published her first novel, *Almost Night.* For her book *Chefs of the Triangle,* she interviewed more than thirty top local chefs, compiling their stories as well as their secret recipes.

All during her professional life, Prospero has dealt with multiple sclerosis, adjusting and adapting to the limitations that come with this neuromuscular disease. Because of her own need for simplified methods of leading a healthy life, *Even You Can Be Healthy!* is a book that will be useful to many parts of society. Prospero remains as healthy as she is because she lives the kind of life she writes about. In other words, the book has been thoroughly tested!

CPSIA information can be obtained at www.ICGtesting.com
Printed in the USA
BVOW07s1102110913

330909BV00002B/7/P